MW00944867

HEAL YOURSELF;
"FOR GOD'S SAKE"

VOLUME ONE

A Physical Therapist quietly asks; "Why do some people heal, but others don't?"

And God softly answers; "I would that everyone is healed!"

BODY, MIND, AND SPIRIT

BY PETER
COLLA

By Peter Colla

Heal Yourself
"For God's Sake"
Volume One

By Peter Colla

A Physical Therapist's Instructional Guide to Overcome Injuries, Obtaining Healing, Health, and Wellness As Promised to All of Us by God

ISBN: 9781790577408

Peter Colla

CONTENTS

ACKNOWLEDGMENTS

I would first like to thank God for the unfathomable blessings He has given me my whole life, today, and forever, as well as the honor of speaking into the lives of His precious children with my own feeble attempts to aid in their own healing process. I would like to thank my wife Anna, truly the muse in my life when it comes to examining, understanding, lifting up, and expressing all the creative gifts God has given me, she is the embodiment of love and beauty being a driving force of inspiration to me every moment since the day we met. Finally, I would like to thank the many teachers and mentors such as Peter Laue and Garvey Graves, who have inspired me to always seek God, especially in the health care environment. They, among the countless others, whom through their own search for truth, real healings, and treatments, discussions of faith and sacrifice could be recognized not only in these pages but also in the written accounts of the greatest healer to ever be spoken of; Jesus. It is in the eyes and testimonies of the many hundreds of people I had interacted in my own healing education throughout my whole life, that these truths were revealed.

Introduction; What If?

What if healing is available to everyone around us, given freely and completely without fear or the need to worry whether or not someone might have enough money to pay for it? Why should it cost something at all, was the knowledge not given freely to our fathers and mothers, or theirs before them?

What if a thought was directed towards the "cause" of problems as a direction of treatment, or a possible cure, rather than primarily directed to the elevation of symptoms, and merely the effects of sicknesses and injuries?

If healing, like blessings, is promised to all, rained down on us all like the independent drops that fall on all the children's heads regardless of who they are or how much money or status they possess, shouldn't healing thus be the same, and realizing this, free obtainable for everybody, wouldn't the world be a better place?

If we may suppose, sicknesses are merely storms that each of us must endure in order to overcome in our lives, having the potential to progress us from one place to another, a better place, a stronger place, a new place, a clean place, we might actually thank God for these storms because without the winds that they possess we might not have the ability to get to the other side?

A person can find themselves on such a journey sometimes hardly knowing the ship has sailed. Little do we know, that we may have stepped casually from one stepping stone to another, daydreamers walking along the gangplanks of gardens, finding ourselves suddenly aboard a ship whose destinations unknown makes us little more than unaware stowaways wondering onto valiant voyage destined for distant shores yet unknown and undiscovered growth. Who knows maybe the secret to the God gene awaits like some lost fountain of youth just within for an unexacting child to but turn over the right stone to reveal the golden nugget below?

What if today is such a day, for me, for us, because in and around the not so random steps of broader expanses of realization, thoughts of healing begin to find their way into the subtle dispositions of one's mind?

I guess I was on a journey to discover health, maybe healing, no truth.

What if we have been given in each and every one of our lives, everything we need in which to overcome any and all sicknesses or injuries we might find ourselves facing, but all we have to do is pick up the tools and use them, would we venture another look?

Is it not said; "You have not because you ask not?"

So what if this particular day is such a day? So I asked....

"Why do some people get better and others don't?"

"I would that everyone is healed." A whisper, a thought, a causal wind blowing softly with the deepest resonating understanding, softly filling sails of one's mind with invisible power, enough to push the heaviest ships across almost infinite seas. That voice, that pure soft yet powerfully good voice responds.

"Many ask but rarely stop to listen to what they need to do to receive, or even look up to receive the very gift that is already given."

Existing in the health care profession, as many might tell you, especially after many years of practicing, gives a person a sense that they are nothing more than assembly line-like deliverers of meager portions of health, delved out in the most minimalistic fashion to the streams of people coming through the door and stepping up in line, hands out in hopeful reception, like some orphan begging for just another spoon of the porridge, all with their eyes wide in expectation for what; an answer, a little tidbit of information, that may lead to ease of burden, a reduction of irritation, the subtle elevation of the burden carried by them?

Is this all we have become? Is there not more than the orphan's portion of gruel we have become so accustomed to just accepting as if it was all we deserve, being mere victims of this present and clear torment the irritation of the storm's journey has presented us thus far?

And what, I might even ask myself, can you give them anyway, anything a person hasn't given to a hundred, maybe a thousand other times prior to these, regardless of the situation or structures of the facilitator that brings forth any change in the issuing event in the first place?

A person finds themselves in such a present model, whether the healthcare provider or recipient thereof and over the course of so many years being merely a participator of regurgitated leaflets of information that vary if anything from one to the other with as little variation as one might see in looking at the difference between various aspirin pills in a single bottle. This monogamy starts over time to inflict a more questionable realization in one's heart as to what exactly are you doing here? Are they really helping anyone? And what's the meaning of it all, is there meaning, or am I just wasting time?

In such days, I found myself wondering and asking, if there is more, and if so what? Why not ask, and since I alone, why not ask out loud?

"So if You would that everyone would be healed, what is stopping them, why do only a few seem to be healed?" Not as much as expecting an answer, but merely stating to myself the frustrations I seem to feel with the job as a whole. Then the most shocking answer came instantly and unexpectedly.

"They Are!"

Having heard tales of a fountain of youth, a magic potion, a secret cure only known to the elite, miracles that happen to others, a diamond in the ruff, perhaps a God gene whose key merely has to be turned in order to unlock the door to health and wellness. But aren't those just stories, things that seem to happen to others?

What if it is really true, what if we could all be healed?

What if we could take a journey and be shown how true healing can be granted to everyone who merely asks, and afterward how Godly therapy could be, would be, and should be performed on the aftermath of any affliction, just as it may have already demonstrated so many times and with so many healers before?

What if we could take a journey on the quest to really find the God Gene?

Healing

Healing is the most basic of physical necessity, and as physical people, we are defined by the observable world around us, seemingly limited within the scope of what we can see, feel, taste, or hear.

Yet the body that God has given us, has the ability to heal itself continually, that ability while given, must also be accepted.

People like children only know what they have been fed, whether being through their mouth, or in the light in their eyes, sounds in their ears, or the sensations presented physically to their body, this awareness is a combined realization of the total stimulus that they have received throughout their own living experiences. This reality is then constructed within the realm of the understanding composited into them over the course of their experience. It is no different when it comes to healing.

People have come to the misbelief that healing like medicine is something granted to those who are deserving through payment or action, given them through a formally schooled and learned medical provider, authorized by the recognized authority who is certified by the state, these entities are given not only authority over the decision making processes of our care, but the responsibility for the proper analyzation, further education, and implementation of this care.

Thus it could also be said, that this entity outside ourselves has been given all the control of our health care options, and subsequently the control of our very individual health, leaving us with a beggar-like posture clawing for the crumbs it decides to give for our would-be health. In effect we have become, at least in our dispositions a sort of slave to then, basically, even with the most rudimentary decision-making freedom at least when it comes to healthcare, this basic right has been given over knowingly or in most cases unknowingly to someone else.

I found it shocking as an experienced medical provider when realizing that the majority of the people who sat at the position of deciding who may be granted authorization for care or not, had, for the most part, no medical training what so ever, they merely sat in front of computer screens and read the acceptable limited treatment parameters for specific diagnosis codes as was reported on the computer of the insurance company. For the most part, their only job or concern was to keep the costs as minimal as to ensure if any benefit was to be paid or in some cases performed, they absolutely had to provide it, usually stalling or demanding enough red tape to possibly make the person in need eventually give up. But there was always a fine line, they could not delay or deny too much as to placing the company at risk of being in breach of their contractual promises with the patients.

Without getting too much into the political, ethical, social, or even spiritual side of who exactly is in control of our health care, or exactly why this shift has occurred, the fact of the matter is we have long given away the charge of our care. The very analysis of what happens to us, the choice of approved medical procedures, the very doctors that we have been programmed our entire lives to unquestionably trust, to provide us the truest and most effective medical treatment courses, no longer make the ultimate decisions regarding care, they also have conformed to the recommendations of what is considered approved, recommended, or more importantly authorized as care.

We have for simpler terms given away the freedom of our health, to the point where we have merely become complete events of fractional cost analysis and containment to the greater authority, and this authority is not God.

The first task is we must do towards health is we must take

back the decision-making ability in our health care to ourselves. People don't realize that they have the ability each and every day given them by God to decide for themselves. Healing is promised to every individual, promised by God, and since He always keeps all of His promises, we can either believe, choose to believe God, or not it is our choice.

What doesn't kill us makes us stronger, another promise, a difficult concept to place within the understanding of the health care system as we know it, but again if we are willing to accept the idea that God is real, and then keeps His promises, then we must assume He keeps all of them regardless of what precipitating factor we may feel disqualifies us from that promise? Believing we are not doomed to outcomes of sicknesses just because we have been told this by someone else, this action then becomes an active and conscious choice we must make, at least as adults. Nobody knows when they will die, this information is granted alone to God, and to make such claims in itself seems to by nature to be an act that places that person, at least by vanity in the seat of God.

We'll start with an idea, that healing is up to God alone, just the contemplation that perhaps there is more to health and wellness than what we have been told is a great first step.

We are in essence lifting our heads up out of the muck we have fallen, picking them up out of the dark and looking at the light, looking back to the mountains from the deep desert valley we have walked into, or the violent storm we have inadvertently sailed into?

Shall we take a step or two into a safer, peaceful and godly garden, I'd have you take my hand if I was there with you, but for now we can imagine?

Children of the Morning Sun

Many children sit alongside the road and are crying, stomachs sore, hands aching because they are so hungry. Only the fewest bites of food are not even close to satisfying the hunger that is piercing their insides like a sharp sword digging deep into the soft bellies. The sword comes from outside, but the pain is inside, tears of damage these heartless attacks have inflicted on a world, a body, a soul of which they have called home for as long as they have remembered.

Hands and feet ache, so much so, that they can hardly walk anywhere else. Where would they go? For they are right in the place, doing exactly what they have been told to, by the very rulers they have submitted to for generations. And where would they go anyway, there is nowhere apparent they can go for relief, all the teachers are telling them to just sit still and drink the drops or eat the bits of dirty filthy blackened waste they are given as food, eat the black tar that is given, for everybody knows from death it comes and to death, it is meant to bring. But what other choice do they have, do not the experts tell them; It is what is done?

Some of the children even use their hands to produce the tar-like substance, carrying it, selling it, sometimes even shoving down weaker smaller children's mouths regardless if they want it or not. These are traders and they trade for their own food, more of the same black muck, their hands are stained dark with the deed, more so their eyes, for dark have they become in their own sympathies or lack thereof for what they are doing.

These beautiful children all just seem to get sicker the longer they sit, and while a few do pop up occasionally and seem to improve, the majority just fall back down, failing from another issue different but unusually similar to the previous one suffered.

A man, one of the children, maybe one who had fed the others, happens one day to be looking up, not because he wanted to take his eyes away from the tar but because if he didn't he would have drowned in it. He notices something on the hill off in the not so far distance, a glimmer, a hint of something else, perhaps green, perhaps pure, but definitely, something that resembles more of a life he would hope for, than the one he has.

He gets up and starts walking along, slow oh so slow at first, not even knowing completely why he is walking or even the direction for sure he needs to go, or even remotely starting to fathom the infinite life that may await? He says to a few of the children within earshot, "Get up and walk to the hill nearby, I think we could drink of that clear brook, eat of the small herb that is growing on the bank, I think I see one sitting quietly, peacefully, and perfectly in the sun, it looks good so it must be good?"

"Don't you realize the very food you are eating is causing you to feel the hunger pain, the dark dirty water is making you sick?"

"The fact that you use your hands for the wrong work, collecting the wrong things, is causing them to ache, and your feet are twisted and sore from you sitting on them in your foolishness. Lift up your heads and straighten your bent backs, it is but a short climb."

Suddenly and for the few that listen, the pains of the sword diminish and the strength of healing flows through their body like the warmth the summer sun on cold wind frosted skin. Merely by looking up, spitting out the tar, or walking in the right direction, life's blood suddenly flows back into their bodies, into their feet, color returns, and the stiffness with its pain screams fade. The shadows that seemed to cover their faces immediately disappear, no they flee.

Hands reach out and help others, brothers help sisters, children help parents, they all seem to help themselves picking up lives in the process of giving even as they receive. Each cupping the clear cool water to drink, the fresh pure air fills their longs, the gentle God-given herb touched their soul as they eat, and with great thanks, they become refreshed. Many begin experiencing healing the very moment they move toward the new direction, even in the fraction of a moment they begin in their spirit to start to believe they actually can get better.

The herbs are everywhere ripe and eager to be picked, their taste a perfected blend of everything they know they need to satisfy the desires of their bodies need. Some of the children partake of this colored flower, others another, but each seems to know exactly which one is the right one for them. The sun revealed it clearly in the mountains. With each cupped handful of clear cool water, they drink, and they become more and more refreshed, like taking a river of pure water and cleaning the muddy floor with it, the darkness of years of stain washes away in but a moment.

Oh, how they give loving smiles and speak thankfulness for

the water they drink. One can almost hear the soft rumbling sounds of the water in response, waves rolling softly on the shores of life's warm sands. A child can almost hear the soft rumbling sound of thankfulness in the water as it too is being used as God intended from even unto creation.

Each child experiences healing in their own unique manner and at various moments along the path of which they have picked up their mats and started to walk along. The minute they moved towards the new direction, ideas, and dreams flow from the mouths of the children in exhilaration as they marvel at the diversity and majesty of a world they only moments before hardly realized existed.

Spirits before that were hardly aware of anything but the tar, sitting in tear and doubt, now start to believe they can actually get better, where painful paralysis once lied, now the same spirit fly. the world seems so bright and fresh, new as a baby's sweet breath.

Many of the young children run back and tell others of the wisdom they have heard, some even bring the nourishment back. The disease that they all were told was incurable, flees their bodies like cockroaches fleeing when the light is suddenly turned on, and murmurs of despair are replaced with sudden smiles and voices of happiness, hope, and faith.

The children discard the black tar they have clung to for so long, they spit out the filthy liquid they have been told to drink, they now know that healing rains down upon them from above and silently give thanks up unto the mountain at which their liberation has sprung.

Understanding the relative structures of why some people get diseases and others don't especially when considering not only the effects of sickness but the cause, it is important for a person to set aside everything we have been taught regarding sicknesses and open our minds to a new and more complete understanding of the sickness process as a whole.

Sicknesses are the result of outside attacks on the healthy perfectly created structures or systems of our body, and simply stated it is no different than basically the results of us swimming around in filthy water, and then getting polluted.

Rebellion finds itself in many forms, great and small, in large social environments even entire countries, and as small as in the very cells that inhibit our own social structures that form our bodies. The rebellion is not the sickness, it is the product of the prompting the sickness causes, rebellion is the reaction.

When a twig is bent enough it finally snaps, it is no more the twig's fault or the break itself these are merely reactions to the forces being pressed upon it from outside.

A Cork Upon the Ocean

We are as unto a small cork bobbing upon the waves of the waters of this world, and as well, we are also the essence of all the waters of the world residing in every aspect of the whole limitless and infinitely created perfection.

Another example came to mind when thinking about this life as it was created. In 2016 my wife and I considered the position of a person as related to the more mind, body, and spirit therapeutic effectiveness, and how it may find its place in the entire scope of the universe as it was created, it was at this moment an image emerged perhaps it was a dream, or a momentary flash of understanding, that later transcended in the discussion as it birthed its way from thought to spoken word.

The world, or the science community would like to refer to us as a most insignificant speck on a world spinning on its axis 24,000 miles per hour at the equator. The Earth revolves around the sun at 18.5 miles/second which is an astonishing 66,600 miles per hour. Our solar system is traveling around our own galaxy at an astonishing rate of 143 miles per second, and our own galaxy while the total seems to change every year based on newly discovered finding and further disproven old theories, the most recent figure seems to be that at any one time our bodies are hurtling through space at an astonishing 1.3 million miles per hour.

What is amazing is that if we are to believe that we were created with a purpose and are truly significant then how does that fit in the infinite spectrum of the universe? Perhaps we must reconsider the actual small reality of what science would call our actual physicality.

Let us take a common example of the basketball size atom nucleus of hydrogen, the single electron would only be smaller than a ping pong ball and circle almost 2 miles away. Now if we were even a hundred feet in the air that basketball would shrink in perspective from the field of vision to nearly nothing and the ping pong ball would definitely be an invisible speck against the distant background. Science says the space between the atoms even greater and all the space in between completely empty.

All that empty space infinitely small specks against a background of space and nothingness, kind of like outer space and the speckles of pinpoint stars against an infinite background of empty space.

Is this not kind of like, a cork floating on the ocean?

So if our life at least the physical being of the energy that represents our body is by example the cork on the ocean, then the waves, wind, sunbaking on the surface, the rain, and even fishes nibbling on the cork, represent all of the stimuli our minds have to process. Basically, our mind comprehends the individual waves and every aspect of the wind it feels. All of these being categorically placed on the library shelves of our mind, for later reference to access and compare to new experiences all good or bad. The many corks that haphazardly float by, how random, how impossible to find another in the whole ocean of floating?

The realm of the physical body is like a cork on an ocean.

Even if the cork eventually is destroyed or ages to the point where it may fall apart and sink, the atoms that make up the cork merely move on to other functional parts of structures found around the relative space occupied by the cork. As parts of the cork move on like hairs on our head fall to the floor, so do the energies of the many atoms and specific everything that takes up any small fraction of space, in the vast continuum we call the physical universe, move to another place in the spectrum of what we understand as this momentary physical space. What happens to the memories of all the waves and sun? Where are they in the aging picture? Maybe just maybe the memories or actions are all added to the ocean like the smallest fractions of drops, some light and some dark, but each dissolving in the great waves, today's ink spots are tomorrow's dispersed thoughts scattered among the fishes?

Your mind is the experiential recording of everything that happens to the cork.

Science or more over the scientists would say that while energy can change its form, it cannot be either created or destroyed and if this so speaks right into the everlasting statement of what God has said to describe the creative universe He has created. But so do the many words we speak, for do they not produce waves of sound, ripples on the waters of the universe around us, good and bad in their own intent or result?

Let us then suppose that our experiential mind or the consciousness of which we experience dwells in the ocean. Then if every experience, every thought, every action, or reaction is like dropping a drop of ink into a glass. By the law of diffusion, the ink molecules will disperse to a point of lower concentration until the entire glass is completely blended evenly throughout and will distribute itself evenly throughout the entire volume. What is the limit of this; a bowl, a swimming pool, a lake, an ocean?

So if the spirit our spirit gets their drops of emotions and beliefs deposited by the actions, and reactions of this life, then into the ocean is like the place where they may be deposited, then what is the expanse or limit of the spirit? The answer; the entire ocean! The ocean is God, our life expands throughout this realm and becomes a part, seemingly insignificant part, but if the ocean is ever-changing even by infinite single drops at a time, is not each completely significant, because they all have the ability to "create change". We are truly created in the image of God, and our every word is significant.

Your spirit is the ocean, God is the ocean and everything beyond.

The drops of ink as they spread out throughout the entire unlimited expanse of this ocean, not limited by time, or space, everlasting and infinite. We are not the ocean, for we didn't create it, but we are part of it as we are created in its image, and thus through an experiential gift we call life, we get to add to it good or bad as we chose in the desire of our existence. Science tells us we come from the ocean? Interesting realization!

Believing is the essence of existing in the realm of the spirit. A person can have something happen to them physically, in one part or fractional place on their body, but since it is with the complexity of the mind, we place the experience into the vault of calculations of memories past, present, and even in the possible future, for analyzation of events yet to come and decisions of whether we desire these or reject them based on the tilt of the teeter-totter the essence of our desire leans us? The momentary real experience is in totality is but a fraction in the effect it encompasses, and when added this complete momentary effect compared to the vast almost limitless expanse of the spirit, each and every moment of this life has on the total beliefs of the spirit, that being said what the spirit believes or feels about a thing or event, seems to be based purely on the resulting repetitive occurrences? Basically the more dark ink, the darker the waters, and vice versa.

If we are truly mostly spiritual beings, and the spirit has the far greatest effect on our lives, then it must also be true for health and healing. Ignoring the spirit in our health considerations is basically the same as a cork ignoring the waves or dark skies during a storm?

The body is the smallest fraction of you, the now, one

moment of one day.

As I was showed the body is the least of the amount of actual physical realism in the created universe only taking up a fraction of the existed space in one moment of time and space. The mind is a databank, in effect a storage library of all past and present stimulus the body receives through the actions and experiences of your life with the outside world, as well as the storage house of every spoken as well as heard word, the every images your eyes receive, and every taste or reaction the food your body takes in experiences, the very dreams and thoughts you contemplate throughout this short physical life which represents your life.

The mind with its accumulated awareness and even greater recordable unawareness representing past, present, future plans, hopes, and prayers, while the spirit, on the other hand, is infinite.

"Ok, let us continue the assumption;"

Your spirit is as a great ocean, vast almost limitless, and as infinite as the surface of the oceans waters, as deep as the very recesses of the greatest abyss, far beyond the ability to seep its most intricate touch, much higher than the highest climbing water molecule up unto the great currents of glorious winds. Within this air, the waters of your thoughts and dreams dance, the deeds and words you speak in every thought the realities of your every creation.

Each drifting from time to time into the heavens, just to fall back down in their own time, symphonies in the clouds of heaven realms just to cool to droplets or crystallize into solid dreams of created ideas that when touched with good and godly aspects form the most beautiful and individually perfect snowflake formations, fall to earth in real memories.

Tears, they drop down the faces of the most perfectly created children any Father could ever hope to realize. Even deeper than you can possibly comprehend in the deepest recesses under the surface and throughout the entire world, throughout every living creature, they touch, flowing constantly transferring their actual physical and molecular essences through the entire created world.

It is as a flowing ballet of created energy amassed into a momentary and everlasting masterpiece of harmonic and perfected landscape formulated for one purpose, to exhibit the grandeur and complexity of the I-Am. And you do it every single moment of every day.

The ocean, in essence, is God manifested, and you are a part of that Creation part of it, not all of it but not lacking any part of it as well.

Sicknesses and injuries are no more than momentary effects on the cork at one moment in time and space and have very little effect if any on the entire ocean, as a matter of fact, the actual events of a particularly aggressive wave or irritating fish have only the most fractional effect on the ocean as a whole.

When dealing with sicknesses if you will address your treatment or how you TREAT these attacks relative to their significance compared to you, you will have the greatest chance of overcoming, in fact, you will be guaranteed to overcome because it is promised.

If the body is the least of you, the mind more, and the spirit the greatest, then the healing and or treatment should reflect this. But in the world, as it stands in health care today the opposite is taught as true. Let us take back our truth, let us take back our decisions of what or who we are.

I chose to share the wisdom I have been freely given, and in sharing receive the same love back in the rhythmic interactions life's gentle swells produce, regardless of insurance and spiritual enslavement. We can look up, we can say no to the waves, we can call out to God; what does it mean, what I Am to learn.

I will let God tell me what I Am and no-one else!

Leave My Body Alone!

How do medical practitioners consider the body, mind, and spirit all at the same time? As a Therapist I have always been taught to consider the most basic point of the injury, trying to identify the exact location an injury manifests, then apply the therapeutic treatment to the specific structures that need to be repaired.

Many people believe the soul to be the small consciousness that rests somewhere in the middle of their chest, softly and inconsequentially pulling them one way or the other, something that is often ignored and often debated by more modern philosophical teachers as to whether it actually exists or not. Modern medicine education teaches us as practitioners to examine and consider, ever-increasingly, the most basic physical aspects of the body as we endeavor to treat people.

There has been an increase of anatomization as well as the cataloging of individuals into regiments of treatment models and dehumanizing diagnosis codes, ever striving to refine everybody's afflictions into the most simple and routine treatment regiment, at least from an educational and authorization standpoint. This has certainly found itself, at least lately, in an ever-increasing area of medical controlled authorizing of care. People usually don't find this out until they fall knee-deep into the world of needing healthcare for themselves or a love-one.

Individual needs and deviation from standards of care take little into consideration as to the specific and variation of individuals, whereby there has been an increased desire by the insurance companies to have a label, again diagnosis code, or name placed on everybody, and thus plug in the corresponding recommended treatment regiment for simplicity and authorization purposes. This has, for the most part, turned medicine into a sort of fast-food drive-through window.

The flaw in this approach to treating, regardless of the affliction, is it leaves the practitioner and patient in a position of chasing the symptoms of injuries and not the causes of the injuries themselves.

If a person merely treats the sprain location on the body that occurs when an individual falls, without examining the cause of the fall, then no opportunity develops for the injured person to learn from their fall can be accomplished, the now recovered individual goes back to the lifestyle that caused them to fall in the first place, a time bomb waiting for the next possibly more severe fall to occur.

"Always examine the cause!"

It is my experience, not as much with specific physical injuries, but especially with sicknesses, that often a person is not aware of the specific cause. The exact moment an injury may have started is often vague or in many cases completely unknown. As early as we began to try to examine the causes and not just fixate on the symptoms in the treatment of people, we began to realize that we were treating all sorts of ailments that typically did not start out to look to physical therapy as a treatment regiment? Let me give an example of this and perhaps a clearer picture may begin to be penciled out as we begin to paint an image on a canvas which by the way is merely blank and white right now, this example we will call Bob.

Bob walks in not needing treatment but as a friend, for he was long before coming to the place of need a brother and a close friend. Bob always reminded me of one of my favorite uncles, my uncle Joe, not only because he looked like him and sounded like him, but also because his mannerisms and demeanor reminded me of my uncle Joe in almost every sense of the word.

Describing my uncle may set the foundation to the picture we may try to later create, and thus give the observer a better understanding of the colors and beautiful similarities as well as contrast these two works of art have in common. My uncle Joe, I always looked at him as a man of which I greatly admired. He was quiet, yet he had an observing nature that one might later realize had more to do with wisdom than any sense of lack of confidence because Joe had none. An extremely successful businessman, but for the life of me I didn't really know what exactly he did, but whatever it was I knew he was successful, because his lifestyle was free of the usual worries others seemed to have when the question of work or career was brought up. Uncle Joe had, at least from the perspective of the outside world, of which I for that matter, in this case, can only speak, confidence in seeming to emulate the fact that when it came to business or supplying for the needs of his family he had absolutely nothing to worry about?

Like I said he had wisdom about him, yet had a direct and almost addictive sense of humor that brought people into his life with warm reception because it was easy to trust the man, you could just see it in his eyes, he was a good man. I knew this for no other reason than the fact that I saw goodness, light, a sparkle, difficult to describe but easy to observe, in his eyes. One might find this observation also a bit strange considering the fact I may have only seen my uncle a handful of times in my entire life, considering the fact he lived half a continent away? But, none-the-less an impression he made, Bob looked exactly like him, acted like him, and even sounded like him, at least to me.

Uncle Joe suffered from diabetes, and while I don't believe I came to this knowledge first hand from him, I believe it was commonly known throughout the family especially related to me from my mother, this being one of her older brothers, but another fact was that he didn't always follow the advice given him, in particular, to the proper diet surrounding this illness and the effect it could have on him. Uncle Joe, like many men of this just post-World War II era, liked to have his drink or two or three every afternoon and sometimes even into the evening "cocktail" as he would call it. This practice would have a profound effect on the illness especially the way it progressed in his life especially towards the end of his life, remaining to be clearly a kink in the man's armor when it came to dealing with this.

Bob, when I first met him, never shared with me any fact relating to diabetes and to my knowledge did not participate in the cocktail hour regiment as my uncle did, yet I think I always knew he suffered from the same diabetes issues my uncle did even without ever being told, I guess I just knew? It was these issues with Bob's back that brought him into the office at least initially giving rise to low back pain and a desire to remedy himself of this pain, as well as stiffness, and thus seeking the care of physical therapy to help.

Bob had another skill that he thoroughly enjoyed, he was a top-rated racquetball player as a matter of fact he was considered by many to be as good as many professional players. Now, this was surprising because Bob was a bit older mid to late sixties, not particularly athletic-looking, being a bit overweight or at least carrying a bit too much around the middle, and didn't walk with the greatest nimbleness often seeming to sway just a bit which in itself gave a therapist at least a sign that balance issue was definitely one of the possible factors needing to be addressed.

But none the less Bob wanted some help with his low back pain and stiffness that was beginning to interfere with his ability to even play racquetball at all. I did ask him immediately how he could play so well against seemingly much younger and faster players? He looked at me with his casual smile and said; "When you hit the ball with precision very low, and fast that the confidence brings, and most importantly accuracy that consistent, there is no reason to run around, I merely stand in the middle and hardly have to move." Precision, confidence, and consistent accuracy, he said he applied these also to his life and business, and they are what allowed him to have a comfortable and successful one, not having to run around too much.

To treat Bobs back issue, we needed to address the cause of the issue, and in this case, it was not only the stiff muscles of the low back, possible muscle strain he recently acquired, or the fact that maybe he was just getting older and needed to resign himself to the additional fact that he may not be able to do all the things he did when he was younger? No, we addressed the fact, at least at this time that he was getting too fat, and this was putting a strain on his low back especially when he bent over to get the shots low or next to him slightly out of range of his normal casual reach.

It was at this moment that he shared the fact that he hadn't started gaining weight until he contracted diabetes, and since there was nothing he could do about it, at least according to the doctors, he just lived with it and gained weight as seemed to be normal for this disease process, at least that was what he had been told.

In addition to treating his pain in his back, we began to advise him on dietary recommendations that not only would help with his weight but also in effect had an influence on the diabetes process. He also began a regiment of exercises that built up the areas of the body he was strong with as a means to relieve the strain on the areas he was not. This was a case in my career while I did try to apply faith in the treatments, prayer, and positive applications of God's goodness and such, I had yet to make the correlation of the spiritual side of sicknesses themselves yet? Basically, we were treating or trying to eliminate the pain rather than looking to the cause. In Bob's case, it may have been diabetes that actually saved his life later.

The back pain went away, Bob got very fit again and went back to his racquetball and even played golf again something he had not even tried since his back started hurting. About two or three years after this first visit to the office, I walk into Bob's office and he asks me to look at his leg which was bothering him immensely. He pulled up one of his pant legs and showed me his calf which was extremely swollen but more shocking the deepest shade of purple I had ever seen!

He told me he went to the doctor but the doctor told him there was nothing to worry about and just sent him home? When peoples extremities get really red or in this case purple like that it is usually because their circulation has suddenly been cut off either by some kind of clot, or perhaps worse a case where their own body starts to reject the limb in a sort of subconscious turning off of blood supply and the limb slowly, and painfully I might add, dies. This is a parasympathetic nervous system failure that many practitioners know little about and even fewer have any idea what to do about? I had seen it only a couple of times in my entire career and in every case immediate actions crucial so that things didn't take an even more dramatic turn down. I advised him to immediately get in to see a circulation doctor and find out if he had any issues with clots or anything? What was strange was other than the leg Bob felt fine?

He told me he had just recently gone to a heart specialist and the guy checked everything and his circulation was fine, but he was going back again that same day. Three days later I saw Bob's wife, she was clearly upset, and I asked her how was Bob? She said; "Didn't you hear, Bob was checked into the hospital, he nearly died, they cut off his leg! It turned out he had a little spider bite or something just below the knee, which turned into a massive staph infection but thanks to God, it never spread further than his lower leg? The first doctor he saw examined it but didn't think anything at all about it, that why he never even got a simple antibiotic otherwise it might have been fine? As it turns out diabetes that slowed or even halted the circulation of his leg also held the infection in place and didn't allow it to spread through his whole body otherwise he would have surely died, or at least that is what the doctors said?"

Bob went on to recover, learned to use his prosthetic, and even went back to racquetball even though it was much more difficult for him to move now with the prosthetic leg than before. We never did look to the cause in Bob's case of diabetes, treating the symptoms did sustain his abilities and even increased his functions, yet when it came to addressing the causes of this attack, we drastically failed. Bob my dear friend, more of an influence in my own life than my uncle had been, died a few years later from complications that were associated with the illness of diabetes, an issue he struggled with apparently for years.

If you are willing to believe that every person is ocean size spirit compared to a cork size body floating on the waves, then consider the fact that sicknesses and injuries have large spiritual footprints and only the smallest of actual physical effects on the body. And thus your ability to affect them in the area of healing has the greatest effect when directed in the spirit as only compared to the body.

Like all attacking agents, they have commonalities that for the persons who are looking are unavoidable. Remember these are the smallest most insignificant members of the spiritual world, they cannot create they merely desire to wreak havoc, be seen, be feared, and accomplish what they were sent to do. What drove the bug to bite? What drives diabetes to inflict its harassment on someone like Bob? Why him? Why then? These are questions that must be asked if we have any hope for true and complete health?

As spirits the dark forces driving the unsuspecting attackers, they also cannot create, so they must rely on the strategies and images they have witnessed in the past.

"You have not because you ask not, you see not because you refuse to look, you hear not because you turn a deaf ear towards the truth."

So what I am basically trying to say is that all people have to do is ask, and it will be made known to them what is the reason or spiritual significance of any injury or affliction? This too is a promise of God.

Did God Himself say; *"if you ask, I will show you,"* but one must first ask, look or at least be willing to hear?

Before Jesus healed anyone the people looked at him, towards him, called to him, began to listen to him, reached for him, even pleaded to him for help for themselves or others they loved. They hardly knew who he was, some may have sensed it deep down inside, but many merely heard others speaking in astonishment as He passed by, calling in hope; *"Jesus, Son of David have mercy on me?"* And He did.

"A child that looks towards the light is the first single step in any healing."

The Healing Touch

Healing is not a talent, assignment, or something learned by way of class, diploma, and or enlightenment bestowed upon one over another, or even a calling granted from entities above, no it is the God-given right on all who will embrace His free gift, like the rays of a warm morning sun pressing brightly and silently through the darkness of each of our night's storms, shining brightly in Gods gifted blessings on the faces of everyone looking up. For the process of healing comes from God and is given freely to all freely and equally, we all merely have the right to accept it through choice or as it were free will.

When individuals are given the question, wondering about the possibility of healing someone, or themselves for that matter, almost instinctive awareness arises in which people associating the thought of healing with the sense of touch. People especially love ones, feel the need to initiate some kind of touch in order to facilitate the process of healing.

If we consider the natural world and look carefully, it is almost immediately clear with each and every injury a person responds almost naturally and immediately to touch, whether receiving or giving.

A child hurts themselves and the mother almost instinctively takes the child's finger and kisses the hurt, caressing them, holding them in a comforting manner, always trying to embellish love while giving compassion, with the ultimate purpose to fulfill comfort. The child receives this and immediately responds, there is an immediate calming of irritation, a relaxing of tension, an understanding as well as acknowledgment of love, and an ultimate realization that everything will be all right.

Science would say the stimulation of the fine touch sensing nerves overwhelms the slower aching pain receiving nerves and the result is the child receives comforting stimulus instead of pain. I would like to also believe the child receives love in the way of warmth transmitted in real perceivable energy by the mother that mimics the spiritual essence of caring emotional love being given through her concern, kisses, and compassion. This the child feels this deep within, and experiences as not only a superficial warming sensation on the skin but a penetrating radiating feeling of love that perpetually courses through to the bone and caresses the spirit of the child with Godly love and joy. A belief is expressed and generated in the form of love, life, peace, and joy, and all these feelings overpower the recent sensations of destruction, pain, fear, and sadness. Light penetrates souls and shadows are driven into distant memories.

Inject love, light, care, and goodness, and the darkness, the essence of the injury immediately flees.

I decided to put this to the test in my own physical therapy practice and began to see if the people could actually feel a difference when I was truly was expressing a feeling of concern, wondering myself if they were aware of such feelings at all, especially if this feeling was unspoken or at least in words expressed by me. The only thing I could think of was asking within myself a simple prayer, such as "help them," or "bless them" as a means to focus my intention while I laid my hands on them.

While admittedly, I am not in my opinion one who considered himself a praying individual, the simple; "Please help this person," seemed to be all I needed to facilitate a sort of concentration of wanting that the person would feel as warmth in my hands. This simple statement as I laid my hand on them even for the most simple mobilizing or reflexology technique, seemed to be sufficient to elicit an immediate and palatable response from the person being treated.

I was amazed at the reactions of the people, they almost always immediately became aware that my hands became warmer and even in many cases a hot feeling, a sort of deep heating experience much deeper and more pronounced than they had ever felt before. What was amazing was for me, I could feel no discernible difference? Different and more pronounced was this awareness, so common and intense, that this sensation prompted many of them to comment, feeling it for the first since starting treating of any kind with anyone else?

But what now, did the people when they felt this warmth, did they heal? This was the question resonating in my own mind? Many often felt better, some significantly better, even to the point to where the pain or irritation would simply and almost miraculously disappear, but often and in many cases the pain would only reappear later or the next day and the person would come back for another of the same experience of relief. This left me with only more questions, what is the purpose of this revelation, and how could it be used in the process of helping heal people? Where my hands doing the healing or where they merely being used as a sort of conduit for the transference of healing energies, and if not here, where are these energies coming from?

I soon became aware that the warmth I felt in my hands was

not completely uncommon, finding so many others who seem to have had a calling into the healing arena, they too would receive this gift, a sort of sign that they are possibly engaging in a path of righteousness. I soon realized everyone who has been healed is called then in their own turn to help heal others, this is how a sort of healing gene seems to be engaged and mobilized.

I have over the course of my years of practice heard of and even met many who have received this gift of "healing hands", some have been hailed as healers, but many the gift was not sustainable, working for some and not for others, this too is a perplexing issue to consider, especially when these same people later come to light as being perpetrators of hoaxes or fraud merely as a means to extort sums of money from believing and gullible audiences.

But doesn't God's blessings rain down on all His children's heads like raindrops being scattered in the winds, regardless of the boundaries, whether they be countries, races, or even religions? It is people who place boundaries on each other attributing qualifiers as if God's love needs a qualifier. If God gives life to any and all of the children of the world would He not rain down blessings also indiscriminately?

Is it not typical with us as individuals, when we have received one or more Gods blessings, such as the honor of being used by Him to aid in the healing of another individual, and then take this honor upon ourselves, somehow believing that the healing powers come from us instead of Him, do we not risk polluting the purity of this gift with our own selfish desire, and perhaps even place into the risk of being lost at all? I believe it at this moment we elevate ourselves above God by doing so fall, losing the ability for us to command the action, for if we command in our own names and not His, the gift will not and cannot come.

A sort of darkness descends and whereby a person either becomes blinded by the veils of the world or remains blind in their own journeys far off the path the light and life healing's gift would create in them. I believe this is why it can be such a great responsibility to take on the role of healer, like any other gift given by God, to him little is given, little is expected, but to him much is given, much too is expected.

Unfortunately for many, especially among the most successful and seemingly talented healers, whether they be spiritual or practicing medicine in our present accepted healthcare system, the most successful among us sometimes and often fall victim to vanity, finding the need to regurgitate the healing event for an ever-increasing paying audience. This is a slander against God, resulting in a sort of bowing down to the spirits that drive vanity, greed, and lust for power. These dark spirits have one goal in their own existence, and that is to be seen, lure followers away from God, steal and destroy the very gifts that God has freely given.

Yet I have also experienced practitioners of true or God-centered faith when receiving the healing gift, whether being healed themselves or students of healing instructions, experience a true desire to be a part of this experience at least in their own desire to support the experience in others. When they admit or merely confess the gift they have received giving credit to the True One they receive it from, there seems to be an overwhelming desire to share what they have received. I have also seen unfortunately an almost supernatural ex-communication though when a practitioner steps as it were into the light, often these same practitioners seem to receive the most denials, rejections, and even false persecutions as a means to not only discourage them but to discredit them.

Did not God Himself warn; "Remember they will persecute you because they persecuted me first"?

"Healing is like unto sowing of the seed, and when this then comes on to harvest will grow, multiply and become bountiful even unto feeding many others."

People who receive true healing and recognize it as from God cannot help but look further into the meanings and the greater plan in their own life for this gift. The evidence of this is perpetuated into a continuation of their own desire to examine creation, there is a sort of lure to it that is undeniable. People who seek light, goodness, and healing for others, seek all of these things for themselves continually. Light draws the light, and for all who seek truth, goodness, love, peace, if they look far enough and remove the veils from their eyes of man-made prodigiousness, they will find God calling them.

That is why one must always remember where true healing comes from, and give credit, where credit is due.

Sicknesses are of the simplest of creatures, the smallest of spiritual essences merely whispers in the ears of the first breezes of a storm, it is fear and misconception that make these such small, invisible yet seemingly giant like monsters overwhelming and unstoppable. If we see these wisps of the first breezes and then begin to confess them or claim them into our lives as storms, is it possible we are creating them ourselves with our very Godlike creating ability? Storms become nothing when a person knows how to step out of the boat and stand above the waves. Simple as it sounds; healing is just as simple.

One thing is for sure "there is not a man who can recognize and understand the place in which he stands if he has never been there before, for all that is new is a discovery!" So is it in the area of Healing, so how can we help others in the journey of their own healing if we have never been healed ourselves, we cannot? And just because we have been somewhere before little are we to guarantee recognition of our own steps within those long past gardens or shores, so distantly crawled through in our so recent past.

But the truth of the matter is, if you can stand here today and read these words before us, we all have been healed so many times in our lives, many times without even recognizing the actual process that unfolds within us. Each day is new, our body is constantly renewing itself, and if we look on the quantum level, the energies of only a moment before no longer exist but have moved, oscillated, transformed into something new, a different place, a Re-New-ed existence. Healing in every breath?

I have known many people who suffer from injuries that occurred decades before, feeling the pains of yesterdays storm's daily as if they reoccur again and again for years? But the event, the energies of yesterday no longer exist, and science would tell us that our very cells are constantly being regenerated, in essence being renewed. That being said if the very cells are different than the ones of yesterday let alone a decade ago then the pains or injuries suffered can only be realized if we as individuals chose to realize them, or in this case, Re-Realize them!

Almost instinctively we all understood at a very young age that healing can be achieved merely by the injection of love, the need to clean it, and certainly add light or water across the area of injury. Be that a mothers kiss, a gentle touch, or a caring hand, that and cool clean water, cleaning the undesirable contaminants from the area, or bringing the affected area into the warm light, all have an amazing effect on the healing capacity of the young child as cries are replaced with love and compassion, suddenly to realize the bleeding has already stopped, the danger has passed, the world opens its arms and receives again the child to a waiting treasure of life touches, love, light, and creation.

While people can clearly and distinctly remember moments of the love of the past, trying to remember the pain or exactly how it felt is much more difficult, why? Maybe it is because pain is merely a warning of the imminent attack, being signals or signs and not the events themselves, and as mere signs lack definition, reality, and substance. In conclusion, pain is not a substantial entity but merely a signal of other outside attacking events. And if the pain is not a real event then we can make the correlation that it is not real, but imagine!

All good things come from God, and I believe we can all agree that pain does not feel good, and while the signals for the waning of attack is good, the ongoing sustained and accepted pain sensation without contemplating a turning off of pain as a possible ideology is not of God. So if all good things come from God then logically every real thing is from God and every non-godly then must be unreal or a lie. Not so unlike maybe a shadow or a whisper of a dark spirit?

Peter Colla

Babies of Dusk's Love

Beckoning the evening's air, in wisps of a cool and uncaring grasp, shudders in their later shadows among the whimpers of brothers and sisters, they cling softly unto any resemblances of mothers touch as they wait silently for yet another morsel of touch, love, an acknowledgment that they exist.

It has been determined from the tragedy that presents itself in the form of large orphanages in Eastern Europe, that groups of young babies are often left for days even weeks without a single loving touch, the result is that a child, even though fed, often grows in an under-developed state, to the point of completely and irreversibly inhibited, many often dying before coming even to a few months of age. The newborn child seems to need love as much as any food, warmth, or water source.

A soft gentle word, tender touches result in increase beauty and health, while torment and insult result in scar and blemish. Case in point a few years ago in my treating I came across a woman who for years had been tormented first by teachers, family, and even later by the very men that were supposed to love her, all proclaiming her less than common look. We will call her April, and while her spirit never gave up the pursuit of sweetness and purity, her own self-image had long let go of any view of herself as anything but repulsive.

Through the most unusual set of circumstances, she found herself befriending a blind man who fell immediately and completely in love with only her voice, and in just the course of six months she utterly and completely transformed into the most radiant and beautiful woman, for it appeared not a day or a moment would pass in which this man didn't compliment her on each and every aspect of her existence. They soon married, and one day I casually asked the man in private exactly what he saw in her so early in their relationship, was it her voice, her gentle nature, her obvious love in her words for him, for I myself was searching for such love?

He quietly said; "none of these things, for while I cannot see, I am not blind," for he had met many women, and all almost immediately formed an image in his mind as real as any actual vision he had earlier in life. "The moment I laid eyes on April I saw she was the most beautiful woman I had ever seen, and telling her it each and every day became as natural as recognizing a beautiful sunset or newborn child's smile."

Our bodies have a seemingly inherent ability to absorb and process the physical stimuli that the world feeds it, whether that be complementary or detrimental, all leaving even the slightest fraction of effect on the very DNA. Science has already proven that our very genes can, not only be activated but altered with stimulus both good and for bad.

Children, fortunately, by lack of experiential assembly, are not responsible for their own actions, being literally fed every single morsel of life whether good or bad from another source other than their own hand until they come to the age of accountability. This fact like healing places a huge responsibility on the people's shoulders who chose to take this responsibility onto themselves, the parents, teachers, doctors, priests, and healers. For is it not written; "It would be better for you put a millstone around your neck and cast yourself into the abyss, then to cause one of these little ones to fall"?

We owe it to ourselves to bathe our very genes in goodness, truth, love, light, and peace. We owe it to ourselves to bathe our children only in light, love, goodness, uplifting and positive words, images, and touches. And since we are all called to come to God as children, then consequentially we owe it to ourselves to do the same to ourselves and every living being around us.

"Love your neighbor as yourself"

Firemen or Water

Sometimes I like to compare "Healers" to firemen, these being people who put out the fires of our lives, and I guess if one believes a doctor, a therapist, a priest, or a pill, even a particular procedure for that matter, actually heals someone then perhaps they are? Perhaps?

Standing in front of a raging blaze one cannot but become transfixed by the awesome destructive power of the flames. There is such power in the flames as it burns with bright and radiating intensity, waves of dancing heated motion undulating in an almost live rhythm that mimics a spiritual motion breathing in various cascading hues of intense light and heat. A person is easily drawn into the seductive sirens call of voices just under the levels of awareness whispering almost begging you to step closer, it is no wonder that within flames people have been known to also become addicted.

The intense dance of reactants bringing often two components together; a reactant in this case the apartment complex filled with wood, cloth, gasses, and other accelerants, and heat in the form of an igniting agent such as flame, spark, lightning, or some ill forgotten and ignored heater, results in a massive and accelerating transformation of matter from one state to another; one a useful home filled with memories, joyous gifts, and useful accumulations, to become a fierce blaze of heat and light along with a resulting pile of char and ash.

Thank God for the Firemen and the knowledge they have learned and practice in their attempts to combat these ferocious battlefields. They direct their water hoses with such accuracy that not only the flames are extinguished but the materials that are in the process of combusting are dowsed to prevent further combustion with a true chance for the fire to be extinguished not for just a moment but moving forward. Trying first to arrest the active process while penetrating to the cause of perpetuating flames to further reduce ongoing and ultimate total devastation.

But who actually puts out the fire, who should get the credit for the heroic and wondrous achievement? Does the fireman alone, for without the fire hose an exact delivery would not be possible? A thousand firemen standing before a blazing inferno have no effect if they have no fire hoses to use. But what good is the fire hose without the water source; a water truck or fire hydrant must be located to access available water sources, so in preparation for a source of available water, the city planners who brought the hydrants into close proximity, should they be given the credit? Perhaps these long-forgotten city planners should get the credit for the heroic results decades after their writings were first penned?

But no, without the water in the pipes, without the water, no fires, or at least most of them would not be able to be ever extinguished. In days of old, in places where no available water was or is near, the only hope people would have is hoping even praying for the rain to deliver them almost miraculously from the destructive anger of the flames.

So really who should get the credit for the ability to extinguish such a destructive onslaught; the fireman, the hose, the hydrant, no the water, or at least the One who provided the knowledge in the first place for the strategies, insight, and useful application of such a substance He so abundantly provided to everyone for the alleviation of such attacks.

I guess the fireman himself doesn't put out anything, the real extinguishing of the fire comes from the water, yes I guess healers really are no different than firemen!

Healing could be described as simply as an image of a Fireman and a Hose?

Like fire, when sickness or injury first occurs it attacks the homes we call our bodies, or better yet our whole existence, our soul. For do these events such an accident, a fall, a break, an infection, have lasting effects not only on our bodies but on our memories, experiences, even dreams of a life yet to come, do they not have a very effect on the way we see the world, or very belief, maybe even ultimately in a choice of whether or not one might even believe in the very existence of God?

Yet, such a potentially catastrophic event can come from such a small and insignificant start, a destructive event, or small spark of a flame, once occurring can in itself ignite into a chain of events that can destroy an entire house.

It is no different in the houses we call our souls, of which fires often start by our own hand, by the paths we walk or others take us down, events in and out of our control, hatreds, even unhealthy thoughts, all being brought into our lives one spoon at a time. These flammables can then be sparked at the onset of a storm irrupting into a blaze of virtually uncontrollable destruction.

Wise firemen, some may call them doctors of the flames, are called, and first direct their efforts to help anyone they can out of the blaze. Is not the next immediate action is to douse the blaze with water, drowning the fire, in essence suffocating the destructive nature of the flame with life-giving waters, and ultimately hoping to contain the destruction, and ultimately save the house? I have yet to see a fireman throw oil onto a raging blaze?

If we attempt to analyze this fire as a parable and compare it to the sickness process, are the firemen in your opinion the healers? One might assume so because, without their learned skills and practical application of firefighting, the blaze would have certainly destroyed the entire structure, and possibly killed the innocent inhabitants.

But no, as I said above the doctors do not put out the fire, any more than the fire hoses do, they are merely instruments of the wisdom of the actual gift which is the water. Did I say, doctors, oh I meant to say, firemen?

Without the water, you could have a thousand firemen standing there waving hoses at the blaze and nothing would happen. Without God, you could feed a person every pill in the world, perform every procedure, wave this hose, turn on that fire hydrant, if the healing does not flow through the hose, the fire just burns.

When men try to heal without giving acknowledgment to Him who healing comes or at least seek the source of that knowledge, it is like a fireman going to a fire without a water source.

But the fire is not the disease either. The fire is merely the resulting symptoms or byproducts coming from the accumulation of flammable or vulnerable materials in the vicinity of the spark and the resulting damage caused by the small spark. Dowse a garden with water and it doesn't matter how many lightning strikes it will not catch fire!

As we walk down the paths of our soul, we bring in all sorts of energies into our houses through the many doors and windows of our crystal clear golden glass walls we receive upon the day of our conception or as some may believe the day of our birth, our soul that represents our life, it has been called a mansion of many rooms.

Healing is merely one of many of these treasures we gather either to pass on to others or hold onto for ourselves or both.

For those who chose to look only onto light and love and godliness, these energetic treasures are drenched in the waters of everlasting health and life. But for those who chose the shadows these treasures you choose to gather are embedded in death and the dark oils that burn hot when sparked into destruction.

In the therapeutic process if we wish to effectively fight the process first we must increase as many water-infused energies we can into our houses, but if a fire does occur we must drown it. Would not water be a good choice?

The spark is the disease, small, almost insignificant, and nothing more than a momentous event in a single fraction of time, like a shot of the gun that starts the race! At the very earliest moment, an attack occurs that is the moment of the greatest effectiveness for victory with minimum damage. And yes, the less accumulated flammables one has the less likely a fire will irrupt when the little flame occurs.

Water is the truest blessing in every form, in every possible process, in every solution, especially when it comes to Health and Wellness.

Did God Himself not say; "I am the Water of Life" "I AM"?

Water seems to be the essence of everything that is good, natural, or perfect when examining the health and wellness relating to people. The deeper I seem to investigate various ways to apply a treatment the more apparent the use of water becomes instrumental in this process.

Even earliest in my career, I recall one of the best Doctors I had ever had the pleasure of knowing Dr. Mike, the true embodiment of goodness in a doctor, a real classic family doctor, the picture-perfect country doctor in all of these images love and care. A man I would often see spend his lunch at his desk calling the patients he saw the day before just to find out how they were doing after coming in. He really cared about people.

One day I presented myself to him with some cut or abrasion and he cleaned the wound with water, told me to "let the cut have some fresh air and light and only bandage it when I thought I might expose it to contaminants." I remember asking should I not use alcohol or other germ-killing washes that I had myself been taught to use? He merely smiled and said; "Alcohol kills cells, and many of those chemicals they would have you put on a wound do the same, water is the best cleaning agent in the world and the best thing for washing away germs."

In the natural so is it always demonstrated, as it is in the supernatural.

"Rivers of Life" so did Jesus, the greatest reported healer in the history of the world, speaking of Himself, the Message, the Word, as He spoke of spreading the good news through the people.

His first miracle as reported by His followers was the turning of water into wine. He took something common, something essential, and converted it into something valuable, pleasurable, something to be consumed, something red.

As it was in the beginning so must it be at the end, one of the last events He also performed was using the wine to symbolize His blood. The wine was involved in His first miracle and at the end as in the final supper, wine plays an intricate role. Wine the representation of His blood. He said specifically; "When You drink, think of me."

Blood is almost completely made up of water, as so is wine, but not quite pure. It has an essence of other things mixed in that make the blood what it needs to be in order for it to give life. A small amount of hemoglobin which is a fascinatingly complex molecule, a carbon-based structure with key points of Iron, this molecule has an enormous capacity to bind with oxygen and deliver life. It is all the other things in the water that gives it the ability to perform the various duties we need, or is this perhaps not quite so?

Water has a greater function in the kingdom than I believe we can ever comprehend. Water is used for cleansing, not only the body but also the entire world as in the flood. Water is necessary for almost every vital function in our body. Our body is almost entirely composed of water, and when all water is eliminated as in cremation only a small amount of substance is actually left. We will die of lack of water long before we die of lack of anything else. Water seems to be the key element of life.

Science would tell us that we all come from the oceans, and thus from water, but I believe this world is merely a representation of our body and as we are primarily made up of water, the majority of the earth's surface is also either covered with or retains in its water in one form or another. Recently I heard it reported that scientists have determined that there actually may be more water below the surface than above, which seems incomprehensible since the oceans are so vast.

In my education overseas, one of the areas of study was alternative medical studies, namely homeopathy.

Homeopathy is a particularly interesting form of medicine, finding its foundations preempting the pharmaceutical medical industry we find ourselves engulfed in today, by at least two or three thousand years. It has been written in the time of Hippocrates, regarding the ability of "likes curing likes".

Without getting too much into the philosophical or even into medical physiology, the premise is that when you significantly dilute compounds, the resulting compounds can be used to cure the problems caused by the original stronger compounds. For example, arsenic poisoning is treated and cured by giving the patient compounds that have supposedly extremely slight amounts of arsenic in them.

When I was in Europe we had an opportunity to examine not only this process but also samples of these products. I had even on occasion the opportunity to receive homeopathic remedies prescribed right along with the regular pharmaceuticals, and I must admit the healing process not only was faster but often with fewer side effects and downtime.

The process goes something like this; they take the particular poison, compound, or substance; arsenic, snake venom, gold, mercury, whatever they happen to want to make into a homeopathic compound, they dissolve it in either pure water or alcohol and then press and sift it to remove solids or impurities.

They then draw out a single drop of the resulting liquid, and place it in a vat, a huge container containing maybe a thousand gallons or so of pure water, an extremely large barrel! This is then thoroughly mixed and a single drop is again drawn out, placed into another vat with water, this process is repeated four to seven times depending on the compound, ending in a final vat of water with what science would say, contains nothing of the original compound, not even a trace.

Yet the resulting water is then drawn out and placed in small vials and distributed to patients who suffer from various particular sicknesses, they take a number of these drops under the tongue, resulting in a cure, and this treatment had been used, the success I might add, for at least the last two thousand years.

I don't know how it is possible, but when we as students tried drops from the various vials, a person could distinctly taste a flavor or essence of the original compound. Each vial had a different distinct taste!

Arsenic being the one I tried, I could really taste the specific almond-like flavor, that is typically found in arsenic poisoning, or at least an after smell in my nose, after tasting the drops, even though I knew that this compound had been diluted to a billionth or maybe even many billions of its original strength.

But I also know that as you continually make half of something even a billion times there is still a small piece left, even a trillion times make something a half or a tenth or a hundredth, there is still a little bit of that ever so small amount left.

The study of Homeopathy would say that a sort of energy exchange is passed into the water from the essence of the compound, and no matter how much you dilute it something from the original is passed through the pure water. The pure water has a property about it that sort of draws out some of the essences of whatever is placed in it and disperses it throughout its entirety, thus the significant cleaning ability of water.

Water makes us clean! Water can purify, sounds Godly to me.

Let us suppose that this is true, science today can only attempt to explain through a theory of unobserved belief the many energies that not only hold the molecules together, and even surround the various atoms, making them independent of others, though they also know vast distances compared to their individual sizes separate the fractions from their other parts in atoms or molecule.

So if we suppose there is an energy that surrounds and holds these compounds, molecules, and atoms together and makes them into the significant essence they are today, this un-measurable, unexplainable, and even unfathomable energy, (again sounds kind of Godly) is definitely strong and indestructible, being able to be split but not destroyed, then why is it not conceivable that this powerful energy could have an effect on the surrounding like energies it comes in contact with? Energy cannot be destroyed only transferred! Hey, scientists say that not me!

And because we do further suppose that this energy cannot be destroyed, it can only be transferred as science would teach us, energies of such strength and significance that even just splitting themselves release forces that can topple cities as demonstrated at Hiroshima. These yet unknown, un-measurable, unseen, unfelt, only believed to be real by the faith of the observer energies, again seems Godly? These energies clearly demonstrate some kind of interaction as seen in homeopathy, well this raises all kinds of questions?

If all of this is true, and I have no reason to believe otherwise, then one other fact is true; Jesus's blood was shed, his side was pierced and water gushed out. This was a fact, it was documented and nobody denies this event took place.

What is also a fact is that at the moment of His death it is recorded that a great storm irrupted, to the degree where even the many Roman onlookers had to comment; "Surely this was the Son of God," an earthquake that shook the land, and split the great Jewish temple, ripped the veil, and a rain-drenched the land?

But even if it didn't rain we know he was beaten almost unrecognizable, also documented! A great deal of blood. You would suppose that the area where whipping occurs would have to be washed, eventually! More mixing and washing away of the blood?

Any rain or water would mix with his blood, if but a few drops, by all accounts, tell us there was a great deal of blood and a great deal of liquid that ushered forth from His side. This, in turn, could flow over the land or soak into the ground, not destroyed only move, it would assuredly find its way into the water table eventually, which in turn would find its way to the stream, later rivers, and eventually, the ocean, where it would be diluted with all of the water of the world.

I guess my point is if a single drop of arsenic can be diluted in a thousand-gallon barrel of water, a drop taken from that one, and placed in another vat, over and over again, retaining enough of the essence of the original to assist in the healing of the person with his infirmity, then I guess it is not inconceivable to believe that the essence of Jesus's blood, the Creator of the entire universe, the healer of all, resides in each and every drop of water we may drink.

And He said take this cup and drink, for this is the cup symbolizing my blood, take it and think of me.

When we use water, consume it in our foods, drink it, bathe in it, wash the faces of our children with it, treat our afflictions with it, and thank God, we in effect bless the water with our words. The water will become blessed and in turn release its blessings of healing and life right back into us.

Dr. Murimuto, a prize-winning researcher and scientist famously known for proving this very thing, that when water is placed into a container that has a positive blessing it actually changes at an atomic level forming crystals that when frozen are beautiful to behold. Likewise though, when the same waters are stored in a vessel that is cursed with dark, hateful, depressing messages, the crystals that are formed when this water is frozen appear dark and ugly. Students have even been able to actually taste a difference in the same waters when drawn from each of these different vessels.

Are we not vessels of living waters? Sounds like another promise, a healing promise. Water, rainbows, healing, love, they are really all the same energies.

Knowing what direction one must in any battle, the cause of a fire, the origin of sickness is the first step in overcoming and becoming victorious.

The Truth About Healthcare

The truth about healthcare as we see it today basically falls into one basic issue; that over the course of the last one hundred or more years we as individuals have given away the total comprehension of our individual health care, giving over to others who we hope are trust and learned, to evaluate the status of our health and then put us on a course of remedy for the ailments that befall us.

The problem is through a system of ideological uniformity and a narrow-minded desire to only address health improvement from a distinct and thus controllable basis of potential treatment modules, people are pressed into a course that has such a grim and hopeless outlook that often a sense of despair and abandonment fills their hearts until they give up all miraculous hope, and give their health over completely to other entities that in essence take their complete trust into hands, and then dish out remedies with no better enthusiasm then one might expect from receiving the billionth hamburger from a fast-food drive-through window.

What if this is exactly the motive for the prescription of care? What if this is the uppermost diabolical purpose and thus the system we find ourselves in has a much more dark spiritual root desire lingering just behind the veil that is visible to the general public, and the ultimate desire is not curing or easement of infliction, but manipulation through control of information, restriction from solutions that could cure, and submission to authority with the eventual enslavement that occurs when dependency instead of freedom overwhelms a person?

There are certain absolute truths that are promised to all of us equally and completely; first among these God keeps all of His promises. This is a primary fact we will need to understand as we examine further the aspects of health care and how God's promises are instrumental for setting all of His children free from the slavery the current healthcare model provides.

I had similar conversations throughout the almost ten years with colleagues, patients, friends, and seemingly with God Himself. It took all of this time to assemble these writings as they developed, many in the form of visions and dreams regarding the true nature of insurance and the spirit behind it, the way people should look at sicknesses they are suffering from, and how to effectively treat them to be healed.

Sicknesses, injuries, and all sorts of infirmities are merely spirits lingering within the shadows cast by the gifts God gave our fathers and mothers over the years.

I would share these words especially the ones related to spiritual healing, and others, moving forward in their appropriate place and time.

There was a time when people would go to the most learned or experienced members of their community for help with their health care issues, and these people would give them fair advice for fair pay.

I can remember a day early in the career of a health care provider, one with fonder reflection, a gentler time, when basking on a touch of soft scented spring breezes felt like willows lacing themselves in the arms of those in need with honeysuckle blossoms, cast their long slender branches into depths of peacefulness, gave way to a view to a calmer reflection of tender gentler healthcare.

Men and women soft in touch, firm in thought, rendered all types of healing arts with actions of professionalism, given not for prestige or money, even as this most usually and almost assuredly followed, but for the deep desires to merely help other people in need. This very desire being the driving force that released spirits into the sacrifice of reaching out a helping hand, a man could find a special calling, giving a sweeter meaning to life, that without, would most assuredly lack taste or spice, a bland dish; unpalatable.

Even within my own years, especially early in my career people would come in with an air of expectation more than that, they would have "Hope," hope that a medical provider, regardless of title or accumulated letters behind their name, could help them with the issues they suffered from, help them feel better?

To answer such a deep-seated calling, when one could see the life dwelling within the very eyes of the many he or she might help in this world, and perhaps aid through the seemingly impossible trials of sickness and despair, many often brought to some in the form of quenching water to the dry mouth of life, one merely had to desire or volunteer to the task of helping their brothers and sisters with the affliction these happen to be suffering at the time. The earliest Nurses were Nuns attached to churches where the sick happen to be brought for care. The earliest Doctors were the learned men or women who happen to be schooled in the known processes of the body, and specifically understood or practiced the treatments of the injuries presented.

Was it not a simpler time, and not all too long ago, when people paid for the medical services they needed, a fair price for the time spent. And while I may be giving up my age by saying so, many times people who were even a little short of pay, might bring in eggs or a baby pig, or maybe do a little work on leaking plumbing in the Doctor's basement as a payment in like, and to this medical caregiver; payment of such was just fine!

It was the gratitude expressed in the smile of a woman when she finally came to the realization her child was going to be fine, or the injury to her husband wasn't as bad as suspected. And while the two chickens or newly finished quilt hardly made up for the relief they found, ever happy was she to know that the Doctor, the kind man, who had been such a Godsend, would sit for many a warm night inside the arms of that quilt it took her so many hours to produce, maybe presenting but a fraction of the warmth her love ones produce for her as well.

But as sudden as a thief in the night the system was overtaken by wolves in sheep's clothing, or so it seemed, specifically in essence by the insurance companies. I wrote an article and posted it back in 2014, describing my own realization and the results this takeover of the health care system had on care as a whole.

It was as sudden as a thief in the night, or maybe not unlike a dark mold slowly growing in a dark damp place, whose dark tentacles only show their intent long after the roots sit so far in the foundation, nearly nothing can remove them. A creature of dark-hearted stealth started slithering its evil talons hidden right in plain view, only inches from the bare innocent feet of our children.

When I wrote these word I was given eyes to see the theft within my own practicing environment and how greed allowed this temple of a false god to slither its way into what should have been a noble and caring practice.

Enter the insurance company, the heartless snake, who creeps in with a seemingly innocent statement; "Give us a little of your money each month for medical insurance, so you can be Insured, or ASSURED, that when you have medical needs, the money will be there to help pay the medical bills, the "care" will assuredly come, we will pay for it and not you! But that is not exactly what was delivered?

I saw over the course of only twenty or thirty years, first people give away their rights slowly and systematically to the insurance companies, only later to give away every form of control. What started out as an agreement to pay, later resulted in the insurance companies deciding exactly how much and more importantly who to pay. They used the payment and media delivered concerns for preventing fraud as a basis for requiring authorization before a person could be treated. Of course, they could never stop anyone from treating if they chose, but they would refuse to pay if a practitioner didn't ask for authorization in advance, jump through hoops, and adhere to all sorts of ridiculous control and regulation.

This too was limited later by the same insurance carriers then telling the medical practitioners how much, how often, what medicine or medical procedure they would authorize or not, and the only people who would become aware of the dark controlling enslavement that had occurred were the people who unfortunately fell so fall down the rabbit hole of needing healthcare, they could hardly afford to complain, just take it and just suffer.

In essence, them taking control of every bit of our health care process results in a sort of enslavement of both patient and practitioner.

This does seem to be the purpose and goal of false gods, to completely enslave people. Where first they desire and demand people's first fruits, even deducted from their checks before they have a chance to touch the money they earn, then make them later beg to even have a little portion back.

We must understand the nature of the beasts we are dealing with if we are going to victorious in this battle.

They lie to us! They want all the gifts and treasures God has so freely given to each of His children, all of the health, wealth, devotion, and thankfulness for everything that is already ours, even to the point of our whole body, mind, and spirit.

They desire to tell us what we are, we are sick, or this or that name they label us with, something less than perfect, something less than human, we are diabetic, obese, depressed, addicts, patients, in their opinions we are nothing but insignificant specks in the almost infinite universe, Unimportant, forgotten, un-forgiven, and lost.

But that is all a lie, none of these names are real or true unless we believe them to be, and take these images, these lies, upon ourselves. I for one refuse to do it any longer.

The dark spirit doesn't seem to stop there, I have seen most people who are afflicted; their every desire, their every thought, delivered like waves of stress, anxiety attacks, and addictions, compound into worries, pain, and fear which always seem to be directed towards or fixated on the issues they are suffering from regardless of how small the area of affliction is. They seem trapped to think about their sore "little toe" every moment of every day.

Darkness does not have the power to take anything away from us that God had given, for if they could they would.

Do not be deceived. All "Good" things come from God. Freely God gives us all good things, and only we have chosen to turn our back on Him, and walk away from them.

Our present system basically has the effect of placing people so far down the rabbit hole, that even when a small amount of improvement is offered, down the hole they remain and merely an existence as a scared rabbit hiding hoping the big bad wolf of Disease may somehow pass them by, this becomes their only hope, sitting there in the dark, damp and dirty, hiding, shivering, and fearful for the impending dread their infliction may precipitate.

One day I realized that without seeking the true cause of an affliction, and understanding the true origin of the ailment in question, perpetuating a complete restoration and thus cure was for the most equivalent to attempting to put out a single small fire and try to rebuild while standing in the middle of a forest fire.

Or perhaps a better analogy would be; to find oneself standing on a small island in the middle of a large raging flood, as long as you stand on Firm ground you are ok, but once you enter into the floodwaters down the river you are washed. Sure, someone might throw you a log or other flotation device that will help for a moment, but soon other issues will spring up, such as hidden debris to grab you and pull you under. A lot of good the log does you when you begin to be pulled under the water by your tangled foot.

The health care system as we know it has become a great raging flood, powered and controlled by the very systems initially perpetuated to help us with these issues. The insurance companies, the pharmaceuticals, the many industries that have made themselves rich, have no interest in curing anything, even if they could, but merely have a desire to alleviate symptoms, with their ultimate goal; which is to make each and every one of us dependent on them, using their products, each and every day of our lives.

The truth about healing is; that all healing comes from God, and as much as that seems to sound like a cliché', most medical specialist, as well as researchers, have come to the conclusion that we really don't know why some people heal and others don't, why sometimes people get sick and others are immune, why bones will mend and then suddenly they don't?

Peter Colla

Country Doctor

Where have all the country doctor gone?

I am old enough to remember and privileged enough to have experienced the true country doctor with my own eyes. As I mentioned earlier, in days not all too long past I had an opportunity to work with Dr. Mike, a small private practitioner, but more importantly a doctor who still treated his patients the way his own father and father before him did; in like, real people merely suffering from injuries of various sorts, looking for insight as to what was truly wrong and what could be done to remedy it.

Doctor Mike actually took a great deal of pride in identifying the issue at hand, examining the person completely, finding a viable solution that would not only eliminate the afflicting issue at hand but also might prevent future recurrence, at least within the set of factors of available treatment options given him. He would even spend each of his lunches calling each and every patient who was seen the day before to check on them and see how they were doing; the follow-up call. Like I said a true country doctor.

Dr. Mike was a great doctor who truly cared about his patients well being, he was loved by every patient that was under his care, I know because many of them told me personally. If people came in and didn't have insurance or a fee to pay for his service, a dozen eggs, a fresh cup of coffee, or at least a thankful smile and a good stiff shake of the hand with a thank-you was payment enough.

And how was he thanked for his years of service and giving? He was eventually strangled by the ever restricting contracting and rigid control of the pharmaceutical insurance machine until his practice was forced to close because he could no longer pay his rent and staff, just to be replaced by large insurance owned doctors offices which treated his patients more like a fast-food delivery drive through than actual people.

If we cannot get back to the "heart" of a country doctor in practice, we can at least get back to it in expectation of ourselves? We deserve better than fast food, we deserve fair treatment for a fair fee! Fair wages for a fair day's work. We should expect and demand to be examined completely as human beings, as people, not just as ligaments, blood vessels, or parts. We should expect to examine not only the symptoms of an injury but the cause, all the causes, physical, mental, and even when necessary spiritually, and if the doctors or the authorizing agents are not willing to do this we must do it for ourselves.

It is time for us as individuals to take our rights back as people, "We have the Rights to Life, Liberty and the Pursuit of Happiness". Health is part of life, so we should have the right to access to the knowledge given freely by God to our fathers, the right to have all of the information as to what exactly is happening to us when we have afflictions, and all of the possible treatment options, not just the narrow undeviating path the Big Pharma companies want us to take to assure we use their synthesized drugs.

If the legislators really wanted to make a positive change in health care, sign a new amendment to the constitution to ensure everyone receives this right! Simple as it might seem, fair and complete health care to everybody, at a fair price, taking out the middlemen who wish to gain by our suffering, but that too is a discussion for later. Doctors are not allowed to own entities they may refer to because this can lead to referrals not for the benefit of the patient but for their own monetary gain. Insurance companies and pharmaceutical companies should also be forbidden to own the companies, hospitals, doctors offices, that either has the ability to refer patients to them or receive payment from them for services of their clients, as to not produce a situation where health affecting cuts could be used to inflate profits.

We need honor and honesty to come back to the people when it comes to healthcare. We need the Country Doctors back, and if we can't find them we must become one in ourselves!

I always wanted to become a country doctor? Not because of the pay, because in the purest sense of the word they don't seem to be paid much, as a matter of fact, many of my friends, family practitioners, or family doctors, would often comment that by the time they paid malpractice insurance, (their own contribution back to the great dark temple), and everything else, staff, supplies, taxes, the list goes on and on, they actually made less than I did as a physical therapist.

Maybe the prestige, probably not, and while they may have been held in high esteem in the past, today it would not seem so, pretty much having to pass every decision they make regarding a patient, by a person sitting in front of a computer screen with as much knowledge about the actual person being authorized as I may have about someone I chat online with located in outer Mongolia?

My field Physical Therapy is the area of medicine I chose to study and later practice for over thirty years. For those who have never had the privilege of stepping into the care of a physical therapist the practice of physical therapy in its most basic form is the application of physical therapeutic applications as a means to rehabilitate or facilitate the healing process in individuals after they have suffered from an injury, whether it be a traumatic event, a post-acute sickness process or a systemic deviation from the norms of function following one or more breakdown of normal bodily functions, all related to physicality or function.

Practicing Physical Therapy or at least applying the therapeutic techniques to thousands of patients over the course of tens of years, and I don't know if that actually qualifies as "practicing" anything, merely regurgitating information I myself was given years earlier in one or more school or happen to learn along the way, all being said, has allowed me to see the relative significance within the application of natural stimulus as it pertains to the body both in the immediate and long-term, regarding the return to normal or even possible enhancement of function.

It has also allowed me to witness firsthand where the application of physical stimulus by themselves also result in reduced effectiveness of the applications over a large group of people, thus suggesting other factors must be involved for a consistent and guaranteed healing outcome that far exceeds the mere prescribed and commonly authorized and practiced procedures.

As I read and studied more the historical accounts of Jesus it occurred to me, increasingly as I looked at them through the eyes of a medical practitioner, that many of the applications of healing had similarities to many of the applications practiced perhaps inadvertently by the majority of the therapeutic practitioners I had witnessed in the field. Some people may call me a religious fanatic merely by mentioning the name of God or making references to the Bible, but the fact of the matter is I may be one of the least religious people I know, I merely chose to believe in God. Being more of a scientifically minded person, I, like many of friends I may call peers, have come to the conclusion mostly by scientific research and study that God must be true, there is no other explanation for the infinite order and complexity of creation that can be explained by a realization of God.

So it is by deductive reasoning that I began to believe if God is absolute and true, then the promises and examples related to healing must be too. He is everything good, real, and alive especially when it comes to medical experiences such as healing, then when He says every good thing comes from Him, all I can do is assume that statement is absolutely true. If some of it's true then I began to realize then all of it must be true, the more I looked the more I began to see.

Jesus was the first true healer, healing all parts of the person, not merely the body, but the mind and the spirit simultaneously.

He seemed from a practitioner's standpoint to be able to discern with Godly intuition exactly the direction in which to apply the necessary stimulus for the more apparent and qualitative result. He knew exactly what direction and in which realm to operate to get the job done.

This is because He understood people are more than just bodies and symptoms, but also the experiences of their minds, and most importantly their spirits, and in considering this, applied the healing to all of these areas proportionally according to the individuals need. Healing them not only in their immediate physical areas but completely as to help them on the course to fulfill their own destinies, their very souls.

One of the first things I noticed, or better yet had been taught by God, was that in every case, there was some kind of action which was coupled with the healing, whether it be "Pick up your mat and walk", "Go report to the teachers of the temple", "Dip yourselves in the Jordan" or merely "Go and sin no more", bottom line there seemed to be always some kind of precipitating or facilitating action coupled with the healing, a physical therapy like procedure.

Was this perhaps the factor necessary for releasing or stimulating the God gene? Perhaps this was the God gene itself?

I came to find out that the action places reality into the healing process, not only does the person experience even at the moment a small fraction of improvement, they experience it in their senses; hear, see, and feel, it is through this positive experience that they receive a physical momentous experience of healing. There is an exact event created, they have been told and it is now and forever coupled with their own healing experience, they thus believe.

If you feel something experience it, and know it is true or real, then believe it is true, does it then become real?

There seem to be three factors for determining whether something is real or not at least when it comes to our individual lives; the thing or experience must be experienced or felt by the body, a real stimulus is then processed and analyzed by the mind, and ultimately believed thus being processed or placed into an emotional response of; do we like it or not, are we attracted to it or repelled by it. It is only when all three factors are formulated in our own personal physical universes do they become realizations in our souls.

Realized equals Real + Eyes, things become real in our own eyes, they become realized!

But we don't have to experience something to know it is true? I was born, I was told so by my mother. Do I know for sure, I don't remember, and while some of us may see videos or hear the story enough times, even witness or experience the same process in other we didn't feel it or remember it, but we believe it anyway? I guess that is where faith comes in, having faith in what we know is true is really true!

I guess belief is the greatest factor of the three. Belief as a factor of Faith!

Now apply this to healing or healthcare.

Belief is the basis for all reality in the world. God or as He called Himself; I Am being the most powerful force in the entire physical universe, spiritual, mental, or physical. I Am transcends time and space, for what you believe you are, you become.

Didn't God say; "If a person only believes even with the most insignificant fraction like a mustard seed, then everything is possible, even the impossible."

These are not new revelations, everything we need to understand about healing God in the form of Jesus has already demonstrated, documented, and revealed from the very first moment He physically stepped onto the world stage two thousand years ago.

Exercise has the same effect, and that is why it is such a perfect therapeutic tool for rehabilitation of the boy who suffers and needs to pick up his mat and walk. People often misunderstand exercise seeing it as a sort of program one needs to fulfill to accomplish a specific task. But as a therapist I realize that exercise does not cause the body to grow or heal, the body merely reacts to the stimulus that is being given it, that is why it works with some people, and with others, it doesn't.

If a person wants to walk they merely have to start first believing they are meant to walk, then begin along a path of belief and actions that promotes them to the course of experience which includes walking. Jesus used many examples of exercise, adding movement into the healing process; pick up your matte and walk, go down to the Jordan, go back home your event is already healed. But in my very own practice many seem to do everything they need to do, everything right, suffering from the same issues, some get better and some don't?

This is because the actual moment of healing took place at the instant Jesus showed up, the rest was the after effect the mopping up of the mess. The person who picked up their matte had to be healed to pick up the matte, they believed what they heard, they felt the results of those words on themselves even if it was but a small fraction, a small mustard seed size portion of faith.

Belief starts a sort of domino effect creating a miraculous change in our very genes and spontaneous miracles occur within the body's anatomical essence moment in time itself.

Sounds like particles moving in waveform occupants within the science of quantum physics? Quantum Physics is the scientific study of the most basic particles of the known universe, their movements, interactions, and in some cases, their possible origins. But how does healing fit in here?

If quantum physics is the study of the particles themselves, healing is the essence of the belief that resides within the spaces between and around all of our very existence. Healing as a product of God, an idea perpetuated and promised by

God, comprises basically energies consisting of the very life-breath of God, and as much must take place within the vast space within them, around them, and between them.

If you snap a dry twig at what moment does the twig break? The moment you hear the snap or the moment you feel it?

The common answer would be the moment I feel the snap, experience the release of energy, the motion, and hear the sound, simultaneously.

Yet science, moreover bio-physiology would tell us that a moment before the brain actually is aware and processes the action it has already occurred in the past, and the time the signal goes from the hand to the brain or the sound travels from the hand to the ear, and then into the brain, is not instantaneous but there is a lag even if it is but the most insignificant fraction of a moment.

Even in the most sensitive and observant fraction of time it still takes a split second for you to become aware of something after it already occurred, thus the moment is over and forever in the past, leaving you with the feeling of the effect of the action of snapping and the two pieces resting in each hand.

Sicknesses and injuries are exactly the same, and as well so is healing, they all occur in a moment in time transcending the very essence of time and space. What starts out as simple events become a giant at least in our minds for the realization of reality depending only on and limited to our awareness.

You only "become" sick after being attacked, becoming in our minds and spirits what we experience merely as the effect of the attack. This can only take hold onto our belief system and become realize if and only if a person takes it upon themselves and believe it to be so.

If we are all children of God, then as a perfect God one could assume He only creates perfection, for again did He not say; "All good things come from God"? And being we were then created good we cannot thus be created sick, but then we can become sick but only if we let this process in from outside, taking it upon ourselves either knowingly or perhaps unknowingly.

The logical conclusion is only we can claim what results in a personification within or upon ourselves, or in some cases as in children have it placed upon us. Now, in both cases, it seems to be more like onto the form of a curse?

What doesn't kill you makes you stronger?

Afflictions and Storms

Afflictions can be by definition placed into two base groups; those of which have been sustained from the outside influences such as trauma, breaks, or bruises, and second; injuries and symptoms that seem to originate from the inside, a breakdown of systems within the body such as illnesses, cancers, organ failures, arthritis, diabetes, and other systemic issues.

Traumatic injuries or outside attacks whether it be breaks or bruises have pretty much been treated approximately the same over the course of historical knowledge; basically, bring the broken pieces back together, manage or hold them there for a time, and allow the body to mend itself, and while you are at it, keep the affected area as clean and in a normal stasis of being in temperature and position. Then return the area to its normal function as soon as possible to further facilitate the healing and a return to normal stasis of the individual.

But when it comes to systemic issues of an internal nature today's accepted practices of medicine for most have very little interest in curing anything, merely relieving the symptoms. Treatments are prescribed to reduce the symptoms that the sickness elicits, with little or no examination of the root cause of the affliction, whether examined or given in the first place. Unfortunately to merely treat the symptom without the cause is, in essence, a fool's game.

For centuries it was believed by the common public even taught in schools that leprosy, a chronic degenerative bacterial disease that mostly affects the skin and peripheral nerves, was also coupled with the slow systematic loss of fingers and toes, that the disease caused the toes and fingers to eventually fall off. But in fact, it was well known in the communities in which these poor afflicted people were ostracized too, that it was rats that would come at night when the victim would sleep and eat the rotting flesh from their hand or foot often taking good tissue with it, and because of the peripheral nerve damage of the deceased, the unknowing victim would not even feel it, merely wake up the next day with new wounds and missing fingers.

So one might venture to find a medicine that helps with the new seemingly spontaneous occurring wounds or the sudden disappearance of fingers and toes, but leave the rat problem unchecked or even considered, would in effect result in the occurrences of disappearance continuing. This kind of quest considering the new knowledge would seem like a fool's game.

Silly as it sounds that's exactly what medicine today does. Treatments are given that effectively treat symptoms, such as coughs, reduce temperature, kill living cells, but do little to actually address the actual causes of injuries, and in some cases may even precipitate them, enhance them or facilitate others worse than the original ones hoped to relieve. They seem to have as little effect on the causes of the afflictions as throwing pills into the ocean during a storm and hoping the waves suddenly stop?

More and more I began to understand that afflictions seemed to come in waves, like a large wave slamming against a ship in a rhythmic and almost orchestrated fashion, these legions of attackers wave upon wave of attacks pressing against the skin of our journeys for one malicious group of purposes; fear, destruction, and defeat. Attacks, or even in the form of storms, I also began to see that people could and would almost without exception have the ability to pinpoint the actual moment they first became aware of an issue. This attack would manifest in almost a supernatural awareness on a spiritual level in their beliefs, whether it be a direct injury as in some kind of force injuries such as a break or accident, or a sudden awareness of something wrong in their body. Even the slower progressing issues occurring seem to also give up the ghost, revealing with almost psychic clarity the very moment we first became aware that something is amiss?

It almost seems like the sicknesses, injuries, or afflictions, the dark spirits behind them are gnawing at the bit to make themselves known?

All infirmities whether sicknesses or injury all result from the same thing, they are the manifestation of storms that occur in people's lives. Like storms, a person must venture into them, whether by their own doing or carried on the back of others that ferry the soul through. In order to feel the effect of said storm, react and deal with whatever changes are precipitated by the events of the storm, good or bad, a person actually has to step into them? I have never known a single person who while watching a storm from a distance or flicking the TV off, ever sustained any damage when they themselves didn't venture to the actual place of the storm.

So what am I trying to say, many of these storms could be avoided? I guess in effect t when we are in for we become storm chasers?

Of course, if they truly are storms, then most of the time we see them approaching usually off in the distance with enough clarity to at least change direction when that seems feasible, that taking into account we are looking up to see the clouds on the horizon? You chose the course especially after you are of the age of accountability. But once the storm is experienced, or upon you, it is up to you how you will deal with it, and this has a profound effect on how much if any damage occurs because of the storm.

There are many examples throughout history where people seem to fall prey to sicknesses and the effects of the storms they experience. The oh so many, throughout the life, we foolishly set our own feet onto experiencing the full brunt of the storm, yet others seem to go through the same storms unaffected? People seem immune or just thought to be strong enough not to so-called catch the sickness others are seemingly powerless to avoid, why is this?

Speaking of leprosy, I was often perplexed with the documented fact that people like Saint Francis of Assisi worked with and treated leapers yet never contracted the disease even though at the time there was no effective treatment or medicine for this severe affliction.

Storms occur, there is nothing you can do except how you choose to deal with them?

Sometimes storms come upon us like a little child running into a bully.

The Vision of the Bully and the little Girl;

To understand the nature of healing one must first examine and understand the aspects of exactly what is going on. A person cannot understand, let alone hope to fight a battle if they are looking in the wrong direction or blind to exactly what forces are attacking.

Infirmities of all types, whether they be sicknesses, injuries, or afflictions that can last a lifetime, are attacks from the outside. People believed this once, and today there needs to be a relearning of what is believed about such things.

Today people seem to take their sicknesses upon themselves with a comfortable passiveness as if they are predesigned with or by some kind of mistake made years before, or worse yet, a flaw in their genetic makeup, a design mistake or imperfection dooming them to pain and misery. In days of the past, we were told we came down with, afflicted by, or were tormented with this issue or that. Today we are being programmed by TV, doctors, and schools to believe we have it as if it is a part of us.

Darkness cannot make us into anything, God gives us everything real in our life, but we do have the ability to created it in ourselves. We have something when we begin to believe we do, confess it in our own life or accept what others have proclaimed unto us, that is the question, crossroad for people to decide whether to accept slavery or declare freedom?

There are four examples I will use to describe the true nature of sicknesses as I have come to understand them to be in people s lives based on what I have witnessed over the years and what has been shown to me; "The Bully, the Raccoon, the Spy and the Hole in the Road".

Basically, these are all the same but for the purpose of explanation and future reference, we will use all four, and describe the nature of each of these attacks and then relate them to sicknesses or injuries in order to later reference them for further understanding of how to recognize them and what to do about them when they have already been defeated or overcome.

The Bully, the first, is a metaphorical example of how sicknesses appear in the lives of ordinary innocent persons.

A child is walking to school and maybe has walked the same route over the course of weeks maybe even years, but every once in a while either they deviate from the path to a neighboring street or maybe take the not so frequented alleyway. Perhaps they are just meandering down the same street they have always ventured down. Along the way perhaps back from school, then suddenly they come around the corner and walk right into the bully.

The bully frightens the child, maybe even harasses or picks on the child, dishing out a bruise, scratch, ache or pain or two, leaving the child venturing the rest of the way home, hurt, eyes watering, nose stuffy, muscles aching, crying, scared and feeling lonely.

Now if the parents are clueless, perhaps disinterested, or unaware either by experience or education they may have no idea as to a cause of irritation that may reside outside the surface of their young child, especially when it comes to retrieving any information from the child regarding the abrasions or how they suddenly appeared, they may not even see the possibility that something sinister (sin-is-there), and lurking outside trying to affect the inside?

When all education has spoken otherwise, even the idea that there possibly could be an outside origin to the bruises, becomes something along the same line as the earliest native Americans looking out at the first ships that appeared on their shores? Not only, were these structures something they had never seen before in their lives, but it is also commonly believed because the people couldn't comprehend the existence of such ships when they looked out upon the seas it resulted in an inability to even see them.

Assuming conclusions of reality can only be based on the limited information people have already been fed, either experientially or projected onto them from others, merely picking up the child and bring them to the doctor, one might say that this still represents a good idea?

So the doctor examines the child, renders a matching diagnosis based on the limited symptoms presented, gives the mother some ointment for the abrasions, even advises the cautious parent to wash their hands before placing the ointment on the child's skin, because you wouldn't want to infect the child with germs that are resting on your own skin?

The doctor might even give the mother a pain pill to help with the pain, maybe one for the mother, she seems tense as well, maybe it is contagious, another to help with the tension or fear the child is suddenly suffering from, a nice full tube of oil-based antibacterial cream, cautioning the mother to keep an eye on the skin and if it shows increased signs of redness or irritation stop immediately with the cream, it has been known to cause other complex issues. And while the doctor may be advised to the possible contra-indications such medicines have been known to facilitate, he does little if anything to warn about the various toxic chemical that the cream has in it. But at least he does warm the child not to put the cream anywhere near her mouth or eyes because it can cause severe irritation or even blindness. Yet with a satisfied customer and a collection of his deserved co-pay, he still prescribes the ointment for the bruises.

Now the child is not as enthusiastic when the doctor tells her she needs to stay home for at least a day or two, for she knows she will be behind in school, she already dreads what her teacher will say and certainly will need to make up the work. The ointment seems to hurt when it is applied and even burns after, how can that be good? Mother is told to put her in the room alone, get plenty of rest, and it might even be good to keep it dark to help her sleep. Better keep the dog or cat away, you never know, and out the door he flies to the next client spending a whopping 120 seconds with the pair, actually doing more writing than actually examining.

The child leaves wondering about the dark room, needing to worry about the irritation of the ointment, the worry about just lying around in a dark room, thinking about the angry teacher and the extra work he will have to do, and most of all the worry about the trip back home the next time from school fearful the bully may come back.

Sickness is like the bully, it lays a thump on an innocent person, most of the time for being in the wrong place at the wrong time, and then goes its way leaving the undeserving child with the bruises, scrapes, and pains leftover from the abuse. The bruises are not the bully, nor the ointment, maybe the idiot doctor, but even if the irritation was to spread because of the ointment, or the child was to suddenly develop a taste for the relief of the depression the pain pills seem to alleviate suddenly as she rests and the tension of going back to school suddenly is clouded by the drugs, one might easily confuse the ongoing issues with the ointment or the ongoing need to have pain pills as a continuation of the bullying, but it is not, they are merely tools for the spirit to use, like waves.

As for true therapy to stop the cause, for the bully, once one understands where the bruises actually came from, of course, one could advise the child to not take that particular path? But also knowing where the attack might come from, we are better able to look out for the culprit, especially knowing which street they are hanging out and when they showed? A counterattack to fight back the bully might also be a good idea especially engaging the local law enforcement authority to ensure this behavior will not be repeated with other innocents.

This is a storm of angry malice. The disease is also not the bully but a spirit of malice driving the bully to do what he does.

There are basically three ways you can deal with such a storm of malice; you can buckle down and take it, you can run and hide, or you can fight.

Sicknesses, Infirmities, Injuries, and Attacks, basically anything and everything that comes against you in the form of harming or hurt to your life, does so always first in the form of a spiritual attack, these attacks must find an opening in your Temple and it is through this opening and only through this opening, an attack can come.

The spirit of sickness and malice might send in a lone attacker, attempting to do harm on the strength of an advisory, stabbing him or her in a place unsuspected whereby attempting to cripple them in their strength. Once the storm has arrived, and once you find yourself in the midst of it, dealing with the Storm, running no longer becomes a practical solution. This leaves the remaining two options; just buckle down and take it, or fight.

Sicknesses, Injuries, Afflictions, or Infirmity's, are all storms, they blow in from afar, cause problems and fear, and in some cases damage even unto death, but for those who overcome the gift of each day is growth.

Peter Colla

Your Soul Is A House

Our life is the accumulation of everything we experience in our body, mind, and spirit. Our life is our soul. Sicknesses and infirmities are storms affecting our body from the outside in. We decide how we will deal with them.

Your soul is as of a house, a house with many walls, and chambers, doors, and windows. God builds you perfectly with clear crystal golden glass walls. The house God builds, you form the foundation early in your life, and add to your house good and bad each day with the choices and experiences you live through.

There are five portals into your soul and that's through your eyes, ears, mouth and nose, and through your skin. It is in and out of these that you chose what to receive and give throughout your lives.

On a quantitative or at least an experiential level there are four ways the insides of our bodies feel, becoming aware of the outside world this is through light, sound, taste/smell, and physical feeling. The light through our eyes with sight, sound for the most part through our ears with hearing, food or chemicals and various organics through our mouth or nose, and the last are interactions with the outside world through the sensations they stimulate on our skin, joints and the other inner movement receptors of the body.

Science would call these the five senses being sight, hearing, touch, taste, and smell, and even has spoken and become aware of a possible sixth sense, a yet unknown sense or feeling rectors that somehow make us aware when danger is imminent or intuition about one thing or another.

It is also taught in psychology that we have the ability to encapsulate our experiences into rooms allowing us to close off more dramatic or painful experiences of our past into chambers until we are able to properly handle them. Often these chambers represent the most fearful and traumatic areas of a persons' life they choose to lock up and forget.

This description is not far from the truth as spoken of in the teachings of the Word of God, except the chambers are made by God and hold the various treasures of the life He gave us. All the love we experience, all the joys, the other souls we dance with through the garden of our life are held like jewels in treasure chests in the many-chambered mansions of our souls.

Closing off ourselves to the storms and tribulations in our life is the equivalent of allowing a wild animal into our house and then locking it up in a room rather than dealing with it or chasing it out.

I have seen it often with people, patients who suffer from chronic issues, there are often unresolved issues that surround the injury they are presenting with. People who come with back pain, whether spontaneous as it may seem to occur, often find itself manifesting with people who have issues in their life where they have problems with the burdens they are carrying whether it be in their own personal lives, family, friends, or even in the workplace.

Understanding the basis of the problem is the first step in preventing the problem from reoccurring, and it is only when they deal with these preemptive initiating factors that they are able to effectively address the issue in a complete and long-lastingly way. It is for this reason that the initial evaluation is so important for the proper evaluation of all the injury factors to be assessed, the causes, all of them.

While this evaluation process, especially determining the complicating or initially preempting factors was stressed earlier in the education of medical providers learning process, over the course of the last ten to fifteen years these interests have been less and less required and even to the point where it is completely ignored stating more of an interest for single isolation of affected tissue, a specific chemical or particular gene. A sort of caring less for the whole person than just putting a label, a single isolated location, or a single diagnosis code on it and treating the injury as limited and regimented as possible.

"Everything that gets into your house either you let in, bring in, or have delivered in through the doors and windows in your house, this includes injuries."

Sicknesses are spiritual, they manifest using unsuspecting and often unknowing agents that deliver their dark agendas against God's children. They knock on the doors, we feel this as pain, discomfort, or fear and open the door with our own words when we claim them as our own.

Spend enough time with enough injured people and you will see this point is so true. When I first was educated almost forty years ago people still believed they "came down with," "were afflicted with," "were suffering from," or "caught" this or that, now they say; "I have" this or that, or "I am" a this or that name of an injury. I am a diabetic, an amputee, a heart patient, a cancer patient, an addict, a rheumatic patient, and the list goes on and on. The I Am is used so often these days, it is almost accepted as a badge of honor, but people don't realize they curse themselves.

We have the power given by God to be and thus become what we claim unto ourselves. Our words have the greatest power in them to affect the universe we each know at this moment and forever.

Jesus said; It is not what goes into the temple, but what proceeds out that can make a man corrupt.

"Yes"

Peter Colla

Justin

Early in my career, I had a patient named Justin, it was a time when I had just started my career and was supplementing my new practice by also doing some work for the local high school district. Justin was a young boy who had an advanced form of Muscular Dystrophy.

For those who don't know this sickness or have ever seen its symptoms play out on a child, basically, the child systematically loses the ability to use their arms and legs, basically, the sickness attacks the muscles or in this case the person's ability to control the muscles. These children become increasingly weak, even the most rudimentary activities are extremely difficult. Most of them, by the time they get to high school, are sentenced to a life bound to the wheelchair, many have such limited hand and arm movement they can hardly control the electronic controller of their own chair. This sickness leaves the child progressively weaker in his muscles from the neck down to the point where a child first loses their strength in their legs sentencing them to a wheelchair, progressing up their body to their arms, neck and eventually even affecting their ability to support themselves even in sitting position leading usually to death.

The children have a particular posture that is typical for them they sit straight up in a chair with the exception of the head movements have very little ability to move at all. Justin had all of this, having to sit straight up in his chair, he wore a very restricting back and body brace that held him straight. It is believed that sitting up straight actually aids them as a means to help or ease breathing or other organic functions usually aided by muscles, the idea is to use gravity to help as much as possible. The result is often these kids receive a very painful and permanent rod in the spine to at least allow them to sit up without falling over into themselves.

I had the opportunity to provide physical therapy for an entire school district in which Justin was a student. A student like Justin while the standard Physical therapy might include stretching tight muscles and very lightly exercise someone to help strengthen their muscles, with him any of these activities seemed futile both to myself and to him as he was more interested in playing games or such activities than doing something that often involved uncomfortable feelings, even pain.

Let me tell you what I do remember about Justin.

I remember remarkably much about him, I remember how there was very little I could do with him, his paralysis was almost complete. No spasm or contracture to speak of, and when I tried to exercise his hands or legs, it was more of a bother to him than a help. The arm or leg would just move with little or no effort, as a matter of fact, he seemed to enjoy more than anything to just play games.

They had a pool table and one of his favorite activities was strapping a pool stick to his arm, and he would after being lined up for the shot, propel his chair forward to hit the ball. He would bust out in total excitement as the balls went into the pockets. After a while, he became quite good at lining up bank shots and hitting even tough long shots in.

Another activity he seemed to like was playing "super soccer" we would call it. On occasion, we would have access to the gym and with the help from a few student aids we would play soccer with a large exercise ball, this basically amounted to the kids being pushed around in their chairs and hit the ball back and forth sometimes into the goal. They all seemed to laugh with such enthusiasm at any moment their chair would hit the ball. Justin seemed to laugh and get the most excited, often he would insist on driving his own chair, not wishing to be pushed, this would put him at a distinct disadvantage against the kids being pushed by health strong students, but it just didn't seem to bother Justin.

While many of the other children of the class had issues coupled also with severe learning disabilities, often originating from some kind of brain trauma on or around birth, or worse damage caused by alcohol syndrome, leaving children underdeveloped and barely functional from birth with mental abilities barely above that of a newborn for life.

Justin, on the other hand, had all of the normal mental capacities of his other general classmates, which basically meant he had all the desires and feelings as any other child, I guess this made it difficult for me to understand his need to be in special education. But I later learned that he often missed school because of his health and this was the only class, at least at that time where he could receive the one-on-one attention he needed.

Above everything else, I remember most the fact that with my every waking memory of Justin, he always had a smile on his face. I don't think I ever knew anyone in my entire adult life who seemed to smile all the time like him.

Yet as I bring him back to memory, another thing I do specifically remember about Justin is that one day I came into work and had a discussion with him asking him specifically why he seems to smile all the time?

He casually said; "Because I am so happy, I have everything I have ever wanted, friends, people who I love, who love me, every day seems like a new Christmas present and I love seeing the present unfold."

I remember clearly thinking; how could this boy not be sad seeing other kids run around, go to dances, drive cars, live, and do things he knew he would never experience? But all I could muster was a single question; "Do you ever long for the things you can't seem to do; football, swimming, flying a plane, a girlfriend?"

He just looked at me with the sweetest most content smile and said; "I have so many friends, many of the girls, they are all my girlfriends, and as for flying a plane, I fly almost every night in my dreams."

This was so perplexing to me, for this boy was smart, he saw the world, he knew the truth. He knew he was getting progressively worse, he knew he would probably never grow up, get married, have children? He knew he would not drive a car as many of his friends probably already did, or have a career, travel the world? But even in all of that, this boy was completely and utterly happy!

That was one of the last times I ever saw or spoke to Justin, he was out again with what appeared to be some recurring illness, but about a week later I found out he had passed away in the night. It turned out that he had pneumonia, and was unable to cough, his parent put him to sleep and he drowned.

It's a little tough to see the overcoming possibility, let alone the perfection there? I remember Justin believed in God, even spoke of God freely and beautifully on many occasions. Why could he not be healed?

I now realize Justin was perfect and overcame, and now I can see as I recall that conversation having with him only shortly before he died when asked him why he smiles all the time? He said; because I am so happy.

Justin was the kind of person who was happy just to be alive and expressed it freely giving back to everyone around him every moment of his life. He in his short life was a true teacher of the gift of happiness.

While others are worried about what they don't have, or should have, or could have, Justin, was just content with everything he did have.

It would appear now to me that it was Justin's purpose in this life to show so many other people, myself included, that happiness is not measured onto people based on what they have, but it is a measure of a persons ability to recognize every gift they have been given them in this life.

This event happened at the end of the school year and that was the last day I worked at the school. For many years I struggled to understand the perplexities of such a happy young man dying, but as I now ponder Justin's memories that slowly drift back out of the locked doors I placed them in within my own memories. I realize that while I found it such a tragedy the young life not getting to do so much, I only now realize the very wisdom and words Justin himself so desperately tried to teach me well back in my own career; that he had everything he ever wanted.

When I saw a life of Un-fulfillment, of dreams and experiences, never realized, Justin himself latched on to the very essence of wisdom in this life, and that was to see each and every day as a blessing, a gift, another day of happiness, and this realization in fact allowed this young boy to live a full and honorable life, honorable to God. I never taught Justin anything, he taught me!

He was healed, and whole, fulfilling everything God would have him experience and given in his life.

"Justin overcame adversity with faith, love, and hope, and now he flies."

The Lie of Sicknesses

The simple truth about health care is simple; we have been systematically lied to about just about everything when it comes to our health and health care treatment. People have been slowly and completely brainwashed in their belief regarding their own health for years and this belief has slowly been altered toward a point of complete fear and loss of hope.

Now, why would somebody do such a thing?

Medical knowledge has been accumulated over the centuries and often passed down from generation to generation. And while it is the rights of all free individuals to benefit from the accumulation of knowledge or technology that was developed by their fathers, particular industries of today, namely the pharmaceutical-insurance industry would attempt to restrict the access of medical knowledge to merely access through their own produced treatment regiments, calling everything else quackery, and in many cases restricting it from being used at all.

Thirty years ago, I studied overseas and found myself

seeking medical help for various issues, and in those days the doctors would prescribe along with the pharmaceutical remedy plus additional herbal treatment, which often found itself in the form of dried flowers in a bag, that I would have to place in a bowl of hot water and then inhale. I later learned in schools overseas, that these herbal remedies had been used so commonly for thousands of years that many of the elderly people of the villages would often not only know of them but would accumulate them and hang them in their basements for use when needed.

Today in the West, the notion of herbal medicine has been reduced in the media as something short of witchcraft used only by crazy medicine men or villagers living in huts in some far-off land. What eludes most people is even today the majority of medicines that are synthesized are based on natural products and plants found in nature, and pharmaceutical companies merely wish to discover a synthesized version of what God has already provided us and then make money with it. What is the craziest fact is many of the agents that are found in modern medicines and vaccinations, especially some which seem to have no medical benefit at all but are in most cases extremely toxic, found their earliest uses in ancient rituals of witchcraft and sorcery, substances such as mercury?

Investigators will tell you, that if you want to find the truth and expose the criminal, look at those who are telling the lies they will inevitably give away the light as they describe the shadow in their darkness.

We are taught that our bodies are everything. The Physicality of where we are right now, exactly how we feel right this moment is pretty much the major aspect of any disease or problem we might face physically.

The essence of any injury can be analyzed and then if the structures that are injured or affected could somehow be reversed the issue or disease should disappear as well. Nice thought, makes sense and it pretty much takes the thinking out of any problem. The tumor appears, remove the tumor, problem gone? Who cares why the tumor showed up in the first place?

Unfortunately as is the case in most issues the problem doesn't seem to disappear but merely reappears later in another spot.

Mind over matter, the power of positive thinking, Law of Attraction, The Placebo Effect, or various other areas of ideology that put power in the mere way we think, have begun to spring up in various areas of the treatment environment, yet it only seems to get the most fringed recognition often being spouted in the accepted medical community as a sort of heresy, how dare we think we can tell the doctors anything, they know it all?

Belief? Well, forget that, the spirit, that's pretty much for the miracle department, and those only seem to happen to other people, often fabricated or just some miss-diagnosis that someone else completely fumbled. Plus the church is the place that holds the patent on miracles and it seems as eager to keep the church and state separation prevalent to include separation of church and medicine.

Maybe this is why injuries have a way of defining our lives?

Speak to anyone who has an injury enough and you will find that for the most part, people can speak of nothing else than the injury they are dealing with, and more so the symptoms.

It is true, I have noticed that when people are hurt or dealing with a healthcare issue their whole world becomes this issue, and regardless of how actually small, the issue is. I have known people who have nothing more than a sore pinky toe, and their entire life seems to revolve around this one particular issue. They only think about the toe, they consider the toe, they look at it, they feel it, they see it, their whole life revolves around it as if it is some sort of dark black hole, and they have suddenly become trapped in its ever constricting and crushing orbit, spinning down deeper and deeper until death itself becomes a Mercy.

The injury through fear and deceit causes your eyes, ears, and every thought to dwell on the issue at hand.

It does seem in a self-defeated manner, to be an almost worship-like consideration of the little toe.

People have a tendency to turn their faces to the ground, the press their face into the muck and their whole world becomes consumed with the injury. They become a slave the injury, regardless of how insignificant it is in proportion to the whole body, the effect on the family, or its resulting waves throughout the entire community.

But let us get back to the symbol of people as we all have been taught.

Like I said, I have often believed or may have been taught in my youth that when considering the whole society the symbol of the pyramid on the dollar bill is supposed to represent us as a whole. We should consider the perspectives of this taught view of us, and we might even see ourselves as this constructed stone like a pyramid, let us take the one off the one-dollar bill as an example;

Our life represented by the monolithic representation of the pyramid, as is so demonstrated throughout history. Pharaohs, leaders all around the world have used this pyramid structure as a representation or demonstration of the life these many great people, countries, cultures have presented, as a way to represent or "Re-Present".

So let's take the representation of the pyramid; in this model, the body is the huge base covering the mass that rests against the earth, grounded and needing at least the majority of our consideration for anything to continue, unmovable and face down in the dirt?

The mind then would be the middle section, less than the body but sitting above directing the whole comings and goings of the body, visible and aware of its place in the whole picture; above the body, kind of like the mind or head resting on top of the body, the director, the boss?

Well, then what is the spirit? That little all-seeing eye that kind of floats above, small, insignificant, detached, it radiates with some kind of detached power, light, radiation, or whatever, and just floats there not really doing anything at all, inconsequential?

If they lie about one thing then are they lying about everything?

Let us consider the opposite is true.

A sort of reverse pyramid image might appear.

Then the body would actually be the very smallest portion of the whole?

The physical body is the smallest portion of your soul. The soul is in essence then the entire aspect of your life in this physical life and beyond.

The sharpest and insignificant point actually touches the ground. It expands upward and outward for about one-third of the evident structure. This might actually make sense.

Science would tell us that the body is merely a conglomeration of assembled atoms, coordinated in the most complex fashion, so complex they can hardly understand it let alone fathom it, yet they are convinced, and it is commonly taught, that all atoms are merely various organized structurally restricted entities of energy, locked in a particular structure and orbits around each other, and further organized in complex patterns that somehow make us up as Human, and for the most part the entire visible and invisible universe? Real, now and present for just this one particular moment in time. Not unlike sound waves flowing like the ripples through a pond one moment here and the next touching the edge of the sand.

The mind lets assume, in turn, rests above larger and growing upward structures expanding, it might make sense seeing how the mind not only encompasses everything in the now, taking all of its stimulus from every aspect the body might offer but also incorporates memory; past, present, and even to a degree that which we might imagine a future, but also extrapolate this information making judgments as to the effects of the past on present information and a possible projection to theoretical future predictions based on data received to date. A sort of enormous library with shelves for past experiences, interpretation, and reactions to be placed for future reference and deductions.

Then what about the spirit? If it rests above and is the essence of our belief system, it is how we believe, it might make sense that it is a product of everything that the mind processes, all the stimulations the body feels at any one particular time, fed up into the mind, processed along with dreams, teachings, imagination given to us through conscience and even un-conscience stimulus and then passed on to the belief system, the spirit to assemble and collect, building its own collection as it was to make its own ultimate decision; what does it actually believe? Does it swing toward yes or no, good or bad, dark or light, God or something else?

If this be the case and the spirit resides up and into heavenly realms of considerations, one might also assume in our structural demonstration that the spirit would go on and upward actually without an end?

So back to health care.

If we are actually structures of not only physicality in the present, but also past present, future, and more importantly the mind has a much greater volume of consideration of the whole, then one would and must assume that the spirit has the greatest consideration if for no other reason then the massive volume of the whole it seems to be in charge of.

The first step in confronting and eventually eliminating any medical issue a person may be suffering from on an ongoing basis, it is first necessary to understand the issue at hand and exactly what we are fighting.

Given the fact that we are the greatest proportion of our essence is spirit then we must also realize that anything that happens to us good or bad in our lives is primarily spirit-based, and knowing this makes it so much easier to fight and defeat in the case of a negative confrontation.

We have been taught we have little or no influence on the outcomes of issues that afflict us, that we are some sort of random occurrence and when bad things happen to us it is just Karma, bad luck, or being at the wrong place at the wrong time. But this misconception has the effect of taking the Divine out of our paths and makes us a bit of a slave to whatever infirmity that may present itself. It is so easy with such thought to just give up and not even begin to hope when we are suddenly afflicted with a dreadful occurrence.

The actual specifics of the injuries are too complex to understand and must be left to the people who have been taught these facts. As a matter of fact, we are systematically being taught we should not even question the diagnosis or prognosis when told to us merely act on the results, and do what we are being told.

Yes, it would seem we have been enslaved by fear, deception, and false teaching, but when a person lifts up their head, just starts to ask for wisdom, God is faithful to give all we will need to overcome any issue we may seek help with.

Peter Colla

Mrs. Martha and Her Walker

One afternoon several years ago I was aching on a prescription to teach a woman how to use a walker by the name of Mrs. Martha. Like many of the other prescribed home health patients, while I had an order what to treat, the prescription lacked the diagnosis, and very little was further given to describe what exactly was going on, leaving me wondering only a little until I actually got to the house.

When I came in I was greeted by a gentleman actually walking with a walker, and looking like he could actually use a bit of instruction. He asked me in and I sat down to begin my evaluation. I asked; "Well, the prescription said Mrs., not Mr." But it wouldn't be the first time I was sent in with the wrong info. No, he assured me it was his wife I needed to see and called her from the other room. Mrs. Martha walked in carrying the walker in one hand, crossed the room with greater ease than I did, and sat down without a second thought walker standing out to her side in front of her.

The fit and seemingly completely healthy woman, while carrying the walker with her, clearly did not need to use it, and even complained about being told by her doctor to always keep it near. I was wondering why I was there and certainly had a difficult time wondering at the first sight what I exactly would treat since she didn't seem to be suffering from anything.

I was a bit perplexed with why I needed to teach someone to use a walker that didn't have any trouble walking. I asked my routine questions are you suffering from any illnesses? She said no, as a matter of fact, she didn't even take any medicines but was perfectly healthy.

I then asked why do you need to learn to use the walker? I asked her; "Is it because you fall or get dizzy," she said no but her doctor said she would need it going forward, for she was going to start chemotherapy soon and would have to continue for the next twenty or so weeks. She was scared.

"Oh, of course, yes," I said, "chemo does have a tendency to make people very weak." "Do you mind telling me what kind of cancer you have, it may aid in the treatment I will give you?" They only provide us with the most basic information when we come in.

It was at this moment that the husband started immediately crying and said; "She doesn't have any cancer!" "Well, I am sure they called it something else." I said; "Leukemia, Hodgkin's, something like that?"

The husband did admit that they had thought she might have cancer when she suffered recently a bout of depression, but after scans, blood test, numerous examinations, all of the tests came back that she was completely cancer-free and had no cancer currently in her body, but the cancer doctor said she should receive the chemotherapy as a precaution against getting what he knew for sure, or at least what he told her was assured she would develop.

"The first time you suspected something you went right away to the cancer doctor?" I asked still wondering why she ended up there in the first place?

"No, he said she has nothing all the tests were negative, we went in because she was having anxiety, the doctors kept sending her for more tests, we ended up somehow at a cancer doctor and now he says she needs to do twenty rounds of chemo because she might be pre-cancerous."

The two people were so upset, looking like two individuals just received a death sentence, the husband was weeping and the wife just looked on with a worried look to her husband, who she clearly had been taking care of up until recently.

After a moment the wife turned to me and said; "What do you think I should do?"

"I can't tell you what to do," I said; "I don't know the tests the Dr. took or for that matter, I was not sent here to advise you on this matter, merely to teach you to walk with the walker."

"Off the record then, not as a therapist but a person, what do you think we should do?"

"Off the record?" "If it was me and they told me that I needed chemo or my wife, but couldn't tell me for what, for an illness, I didn't even have yet, or why for that matter, I would get another opinion."

"We thought about that," they quickly said; "but the doctor was very adamant about us needing to start this chemo as soon as possible, even alluding to the fact that others who refused to take this regiment later developed cancer were cut off for not following his advice."

They went on to tell me that not only were they told they must follow this treatment course to the letter, but they must also stop all Natural-medicine supplements they may be using, and stop any advice they may have received in the past unless they cleared it with him, and if they didn't it not only meant that this doctor would refuse to treat them in the future, it was then that he implied they could also risk losing their insurance coverage if they didn't.

"They can't make you show up." I said; "Just keep canceling and rescheduling, make up an excuse; flat tire, the cat is sick anything and stall until you get the second, third, even fourth opinion, so you will know for sure!" "You said it yourself the doctor said right now you don't have cancer, he said that himself!"

"But whatever you do, don't tell the doctor I told you to do this, it could be my job!"

They were in tears for the advice I gave them and thanked me continually for my giving them such a recommendation.

They thanked me and I left. The next day the owner of the company called me, wanting to meet, took my pad, said I was a great therapist but the doctor called and demanded I was fired. He said he was sorry but this particular doctor is one of his biggest referral sources.

Unfortunately, the company I worked for was not only a Home Health provider, but they also provided at-home chemotherapy directly to the patients and made a quite profitable business doing so.

These dark spirits seem to once they get their hooks into some unsuspecting or innocent victim become ruthless, and cruel in their greedy lust to keep them at any cost?

Hidden Truths in Lies

If they lied about one thing, then we might as well assume they are lying about many things.

We are taught throughout our entire life, who we need to listen to, who is telling the truth.

Teachers, teach truths? We believe that they had to learn from Doctors who in turn are the absolute authority in what is believed.

If a Doctor says it then it must be true, that fact is drilled into us from as early as we can remember and maybe even before. So as we get older the thought of getting better, when a Doctor has said you will not, this concept is difficult for any of us to fathom.

The problem is as a health care provider that even healing, life or death seems to be out of the hands of what we may call absolute, and actually in most cases the whether or not's of healing seems to be more a question of a roll of dice than the clear-cut treatment cure scenario most health care providers would paint.

Recently I spoke with a very prominent Cardiologist near my home, a friend I had known for years, and was astonished to hear him question the very essence of what he did.

Let us call him Jim.

Jim sat across from me drinking his coffee and stating to me in tears strained eyes that he just doesn't get it.

An eighty-plus-year-old man sits in the operating room, with little or no chance for the procedure to actually succeed, failure occurs, and after only the most moderate attempts of revival they decide to stop efforts for the additional issues of this man warrant only the slightest of efforts, there are too many things that could end his life, and frankly according to this Doctors opinion; "he was living on borrowed time for years."

Minutes, maybe many minutes after he dies the man springs to life, and the issues that seemed to have caused the failure of his life suddenly and almost miraculously disappear. Upon further examination areas of the problem seem to have been miraculously repaired without being touched, but the fact that he sprung to life without outside intervention seems the most perplexing.

Yet another case of the most routine repair, a young woman strong, fit, and healthy suddenly her heart stops during what should have been a routine procedure, the life leaves her, and no matter what they do, it is impossible to resuscitate her even though there seems to be absolutely nothing physically wrong with her.

Worse yet why do some bacteria that linger on the skin or reside in every bite we eat live harmlessly with us, and why do some decide to attack? Do they even know they are attacking us, are they even aware of us at all?

Why do some of us get sick and others don't, why do some die and others don't?

This scenario seems to be showing up more and more in health care today and the deeper people look into the mechanisms of healing the more evident it seems to be that we have absolutely no control of the workings of healing, and in fact, the entire health care system is merely engaged with the reductions of symptoms, or in other words; the management of effects of sicknesses and illnesses rather than looking at the causes.

God gives every person alive who chooses to look into the

light, signs to show God fulfills His promises; like the rainbows, they are a gift to all the people as a reminder to us that God always keeps my promises. It is no different in healing when people are faced with drastic and dramatic choices one would be amazed how many look to God when all else seems to fail. God, being Himself a good Father would it that we would look to the light long before the skies become so dark.

It is no different in my own life or the majority of the people I have treated, people, in general, seem to have to hit rock bottom before they are willing to actually make real changes that result in some good and positive changes in their lives. I have to honestly say over the course of my adult life the majority of the greatest and most positive changes in my own life for the better came on the precepts of calamity.

All things can be turned to good for those who seek God. It is not different in health, storms, or dealing with attacks, it merely presents opportunities for growth, which by the way is every given day in our lives.

Like the rainbow, it is a promise.

We ourselves have all seen rainbows of all types when we have been in a place of asking, looking to God for help, and then waiting on Him for answers, guidance, or help. God gave that gift to men way back when He first gave it to Noah, always has and continues today, for those who first step out into the light, choose to follow and merely look in the right direction?

How do we know it is the right direction though, especially when doctors or people in authority have told us something different?

The majority of people do not look to God until the situation or issues of the world literally force them to. All forms of storms, afflictions, attacks, or infirmities can be classified into one simple example; children find themselves either by action or directions at one moment or more face down in the muck. When you are face down in the muck there are two choices every individual must choose; either leave their face in the muck, give up and die, or lift their head up?

One thing I find perplexing is how many times patients have come in continuing the same procedures that clearly are not helping, even after being told by the doctor "There is nothing more I can do for you," "there is little or no chance you will get better," or "there is no cure for what you have," all of these statements are defining in their hopelessness and finality, and on a belief or spirit level seem to be no less than a curse.

Lifting the head up is lifting it towards God, you are lifting your head up with the choice for life, life is a gift from God and thus you are choosing Him, whether you realize it or not.

This upward motion represents a desire to live on and not just give up. Lift your head, look up to the light and you are taking the first step onto the path of healing no matter what affliction you are suffering from.

I have seen it in patients when they seem to give up there is a constant fixation with their issue, an almost constant bowing down of their conscious spirit, eyes down, sad, and completely negative about their chances to ever get better. For the most part, a person even though they may present all the abilities to improve their lives, they dwell on their losses, doubting and negative about any chance for improvement.

You look up, up is always good. Lift your face out of the muck.

Many people believe and often ask the question; If God is a loving God why does he create the muck I happen to find myself face down in?

It is because God is a loving God that He created this reality for us to enjoy. As in all creation, in order for it to have substance, real objects also cast a shadow. The shadow is not darkness but is often used by darkness because darkness is so afraid of the light, it lurks in the shadows.

The objects created are not the shadows, but merely cast the shadow as they block out the light. The shadows are merely the area created space subject to a reduced or absent light, without physical form, unable to harm you, but it is here that darkness, deception, and malice lingers. Believing the shadows are real, we elevate them to the point where they become giants, demons, virtual beasts we are but slaves to their threats and destructive promises.

Belief is so strong, and I have seen so many examples of people believing what they are told, even to the point of experiencing physical effects merely because their mind tells them it is so.

One particularly extreme example is with Uncle Jerry.

A man healthy his whole life, an Army Ranger, a survivor of countless battles in World War II, he even was one of the few that can say they stormed Normandy Beach and survived, comes home and starts his life. Becomes a professional football player, merely because of his size and strength, not the success or fame of today because, in those days playing meant jumping on a train to go play on the weekend, leather helmet and few dollars pay, but whatever; you are strong, big and it's fun.

He lives a good life, a trade of his hands, married, children, the home, car, and dog, cabin in the woods, soon he would retire and finally relax into the life of comfortable leisure he had hoped for, perhaps longed for, for oh so many years.

He is a man's man, he doesn't believe in buying cut wood, since he could easily cut all the wood he needs himself, actually, the very stove he warms his cabin with, better to fuel it with cut wood than to be dependent on gas or even electric, he can always cut more wood.

Retirement approaches and weeks before he sells the last of his working life's home, all the possessions in the city, so he and his loving wife can finally retire comfortably to the cabin at the lake. The woods and cabin have been calling him peaceably for as long as he can remember, how beautiful and relaxed is such a life.

On the morning of the very first day of his retirement, our man's man goes down to the basement, as he has done so many times before, and puts some wood into the furnace to warm the house for the day. The wood was there already promptly stacked months before and comfortably waiting for the winter mornings that just started to appear.

He tries to climb out of the basement and stops at only the first step, because he just can't catch his breath, finding for the first time in his life a lack of the strength he had so often just assumed would re-appear daily as he needed. He calls to his wife, who further calls paramedics and within a short moment, he finds himself being examined in the hospital by a team of doctors.

Cat scans, MRI, maybe they even do a biopsy or two, or not, and they go into the room to inform him and his awaiting wife that he has cancer. The doctors further inform him as to while they recommend chemo and radiation, the outlook does not look good and they think he only has months at best to live.

Our man, our hero, our professional football player, our brother, our husband, our father, dies that same day.

That man was told by someone he believed, trusted, for this man this doctor this learned-man who must know the truth, and after hearing those words our hero, our survivor of countless attacks of death has no doubt at all, he was going to die. He didn't want to die, why would he work so hard, so long to finally enjoy his earned retirement? No, in his spirit he suddenly believed something and it happened.

No point in arguing, he died.

Today for the most part when we have an injury we are given something that will help reduce or remove the symptom we happen to be suffering from at that particular moment we are told what the expected outcome will be, then it is up to us to believe or not. Pills, always pills, potion laced with death, seeded with toxic oils, immunization that contains mercury, why when they have no fathomable reason to be in these, yet always the ones the doctors say we need, we need to trust them and take if we want to have a healthy life?

Steroids to reduce the bodies symptoms that actually are there to fight the issue at hand. Anti-inflammatory this, pain pills that, antibiotics, anti this, anti that. All these things designed to effectively reduce the irritations these infirmities cause, yet very few if any actually address in the least the actual cause of the issue and certainly does little to affect the mind or spirit at all other than depress and dumb down.

So if we have already deduced that the spirit has the greatest portion of the whole, and the mind infinitely less, and the body really only has the smallest and most insignificant connection to the world, then we can assume that if using only worldly means such as chemicals or physical applications it would only have the most insignificant effect on the entire healing process?

"The effective way to deal with any infirmity believe first in God, see, hear, or experience something with the mind that is True, and then act with the body in response, moving down that path towards the light."

The muck is not the enemy, it is merely being used by the enemy to inflict harm. Look to the light, the darkness flees from the light. Add light to your life and the darkness must flee.

Back to the rainbows and my promises; God keeps all promises and will show you all the time and whenever you look in the form of signs, visions, dreams, sounds, recollections, rainbows, rainbow-like appearances of colors on objects, angles in their appearance or directed actions, birds, pets, butterflies, snowflakes, healing, and the list goes on and on into infinity. Basically, He shows Himself in every creation for those who are looking.

"Ask and ye shall receive, for you have not because you ask

not. Believe that you are loved, and as a loving Father God holds back no good thing from my child who asks."

I guess this is where so many people fail, especially when it comes to severe injury or diseases, they are so convinced by the world that certain things are just incurable or permanent, that they are not willing to even ask, or asking represents some kind of false hope for a miracle. The majority of the people who walk through the door, while believing miracles do happen they happen to others, will never or could never happen to them.

I must say I have been perplexed myself with the notion of why some people seem to be miraculously healed with what is said to be incurable afflictions, and others not. These many good people many suffering from the same, also at times ask, yet are met with silence or even worsening issues?

It would appear that people need healing in many different areas of their life, often unaware or worse ignored by their own hearts, and it is in this area that choices are made whether they chose to believe God or believe what they have been told. It boils down to choice, every soul has free will do they choose to listen to what the world has told them or do they listen to God?

Health, Wellness, and Real Healthcare are engulfed and dependent upon the realization of God-given truths, and the application of these truths, within each of us resides the realization of the promised outcomes granted to each of us by the reality of the entire world God has created for us in this life, this totalitarian soul that encompasses our entire life.

Jesus, I believe the proclaimed son of God, and the physical manifestation of God's own self made physical is the greatest of these promises, I also believe He demonstrated to all of us children the free gift of healing granted each and every one of us. Everyone who was willing to lift their head, or eyes, hear or come, turn towards the light, call, all who were willing to but for a moment believe and look in the direction of God for resolution for the storms these afflictions cause us, can receive healing.

Doing anything with the intention of doing what God would have you do, especially in the area of health or healthcare, no matter the situation, storm, or plan, it has within it a moment's Godly reality, in its creative momentous perspective. Subtlety the result is to form a real event in the spiritual realm which is more significant than any physical movements these actions may be facilitated in the physically created universe, that is the physical universe of which your bodies are aware and resides. For the created universe is merely a fraction of the whole in comparison to the physical boundaries of entirely of creation, our own scientists have stated and presented this repeatedly.

Knowing this fact myself, I always have found it perplexing the thought of so much space. How infinitely small atoms actually are, or viruses for that matter. The vastness of space between planets or stars, or the spaces that science would tell us resides even between the relatively small actual physical boundaries of the components of atoms is almost unbelievable.

If sicknesses are essentially supernatural intentions behind innocent and unknowingly used hosts, how does such the supernatural, the spirituality, God, positive thinking, forgiveness, belief, and hope play in the manifestation of the healing process?

Do any or all of these somehow have something to do with the God gene?

Gary and the Cancer Spirit

More and more as time progressed along with the more natural examination of healing and even the mere contemplation that a God Gene may exist it became clear if we were to effectively treat the issues at hand we would have to treat other sicknesses, the ones the person may have been afflicted with before, even long before, the issues they actually showed up with looking for assistance with could be thoroughly remedied. Certainly, once we realize that the majority of these symptoms, these headaches, pains here or there, weight issues, stiffness, sprains or strains, addictions, even strokes, were being basically caused by factors of other illnesses, sicknesses and maybe even attacks months even years before it became imperative that we must treat also the originating sickness if any hope of cure of the newly found symptom could occur.

In walks Gary, my financial advisor, confident, but more importantly friend for over twenty years, and it is clear he is wanting and needing help. Gary recently contracted cancer in his neck area, the diagnosis, as well as the prognosis, was bleak, telling him he must receive a great deal of chemotherapy and radiation to his neck, chest, shoulder, and even jaw areas to have any hope to live.

While the chemo does have a profound effect on someone often leaving them so beat up they look like they spent a year in a concentration camp, hair gone, skin almost chalky grey and pail, shadows under the sunken skeletal eyes, not even mentioning the overall sick feeling person must live with for months on end, bowing down to the altar of the toilet god as they barf their guts out trying hopelessly to cough out the poisons and deadly toxins they have had pumped into them all in the hope to somehow rid themselves of this sickness doctors tell them they have this could not explain the bad state Gary presented himself in.

.

Radiation, now that's another thing, this concentrated, by the way, invisible or so-called dark light, not only supposedly kills the cancer cells, it kills everything else it goes through, leaving the patient often looking more like a burn victim than normal. So was the case of Gary. He presented with all the chemo signs but on the right side of his neck all the way from his face to his shoulder he had what appeared to look like burned skin. Tight, the muscle under looked more like cables than muscles and everything was hard, his skin-paper thin pulled tight over the few structures he had left in his neck frozen and stiffened, this left him unable hardly move.

He barely moved his jaw and was only able to whisper as it seemed to also affect his vocal cords. He even had to be fed through a tube in his nose, because he could swallow any longer.

As a therapist your first thought is "What am I supposed to do here?" but regardless of how bad it looked, Gary was my friend and he deserved every possible effort. Gary was hoping for some help with his pain, not the pain on the burned skin or muscle under, actually he said, he really didn't feel them at all, according to the doctors they were dead and there was nothing that could be done for them anyway? No, he wanted help with his neck, maybe help with the movement, although he was also told nothing could help, his jaw maybe, he could hardly open or close it without a great deal of pain. He suffered from headaches, and he couldn't lift his right arm, the side of the radiation any longer, he was so weak walking was a task. He pretty much felt like he was a hundred years old?

I can honestly say I had no idea what to do with him! I put my hands on him, maybe try to relax the tight muscles with some massage or reflexology, something to loosen them up, some real basic exercises for mobilizing the neck, yet I had been taught for these to be effective the neck must anatomically be intact, basically it cannot have dramatic changes to its structure or they basically are useless? I was taught cancer and at least the effects it had on the body were incurable, permanent, and hopeless.

Thank God at this time we also introduce sights, sounds, physical touches, advice, and most importantly basic prayers, as a means to try to help or apply therapy to people we worked on. I believe now we are inadvertently turning the light on in the spiritual realm even though we had no idea what or how we were doing it. To make a long story short, Gary recovered much of his motion immediately, he would almost instantaneously felt a reduction of pain and increase in a relaxing feeling in the muscles of the neck and shoulders. Exercises were accepted by him and movements he had been told would never come back started returning. Gary started replacing sadness and hopelessness with a new-found faith, and vigor. A smile returned to his face as he began to see himself accomplish the simple "Pick up your mat and walk" exercises he was given. Gary turned on the light with prayer, the cancer spirit fled!

We even went on to advise him to only eat pure natural foods, eliminate sugars, especially unnatural sweeteners from his diet, as a matter of fact, eat good, don't diet. That was easy since the doctors wanted him to gain weight, he had lost so much in the process. Drink a lot of pure water, bless it when you drink, even use natural sparkling water as it is generally a bit alkaline as a way to counter the more acidic diets we often eat in the West. None of this information was offered by his cancer doctors, and even though he had gone to a cancer center that supposedly offered prayer, natural foods, dietary advice and all other forms of alternative care with the chemo and radiation, he said none of these others were ever mentioned, only the chemo and radiation. He was also told not to use anything natural, fish oil or any natural products teas, honey, or anything, the doctors told him it may interfere with the chemo? I wonder what purpose of a task the chemo was doing that healthy or natural remedies might interfere with?

I recently saw Gary years later, and if you looked at him today you would see no signs he had ever had that horrible radiation burns on his neck, shoulder, or jaw. His hair was back to normal, he moved and acted the same he had long before the tragic attack of cancer. The skin that was thin and looked burned now appeared to be as clear as newborn babies, subtle, and muscles that only years before appeared to be gone forever, returned to their normal soft and flexible appearance, leaving no sign of any difference between his right or left side.

He spoke to many people about how he was a cancer survivor

and how I had saved his life, but I assured him, I did nothing, I said; "God saved your life, thank Him, thank yourself for finding the wisdom to go to God with your prayers and rid yourself of this horrible attack. You are not a cancer survivor, you are a cancer butt-kicker!"

I must admit that hearing Gary credit me with saving his life, did change me though, in over twenty-five years of treating people, thousands, I had never once heard those words spoken to me. I guess Gary's words did more for placing me on a road where I desired to not only help people with their afflictions but perhaps help save their lives than all the other times combined. Perhaps it was Gary really who healed me?

"God heals us, He's the water, we are the firemen who learn to point the hose in the right direction!"

The Shoulder

A physical therapist, a perhaps self-proclaimed patient complains of a sudden aching of the right shoulder. Started out of the blue without any fall, lifting injury, or any kind of noticeable origin. The pain got so bad that he could hardly sleep, and even driving, resting it on the center counsel caused aching pain, to the point where he went in and solicited his close friend a prominent orthopedic surgeon of the area to examine it. After nearly twenty in-depth X-rays and a thorough examination, the doctor shows him on the X-ray where his right shoulder is clearly sagging from the left at least an inch or more, and this sagging is placing pressure on the tendons when in rest, that is why it is aching.

"Have you recently hurt it?" he asks; "Or perhaps did you do some very strenuous shoulder actives may be in your distant past?"

"No, not recently, but maybe back in high school I used to pole vault." The therapist suggests. "That could do it?", the doctor says and offers him some anti-inflammatory medication, but goes on to tell him it will probably need an operation to tighten up the ligaments.

The therapist knows himself that shoulder surgeries are usually only 50% successful and rarely return a person to pre-injury levels, being a very complex joint, to say the least. So the therapist says he will try to treat it himself with physical therapy and see. The doctor says; "It might be worth a try, keep me posted."

The therapist really does very little if anything for therapy on his own. Then one day a friend suggests he sees a chiropractor friend of his that does Kinetics, where issues are examined and treatments are determined by merely pressing down on an extended arm while asking questions, something the therapist is pretty much convinced is hogwash! But what will it hurt?

He decides to not tell the chiropractor, Dr. Mark, about the shoulder and see if he can find it on his own. Within moments Dr. Mark says; "what's going on with the right shoulder?" and asks if he can do some kinetic testing to see what's going on. "Sure," the therapist says, why not?

He asks a series of questions, a series of yes and no questions to locate the cause of the injury. He determines the cause of the problem in the shoulder had nothing to do with a physical injury, or anything that was eaten, or lack thereof for that matter, but had to do with experiences in the past. The results of the question pointed to a career choice back when the therapist was eighteen?

As it turns out the therapist was nominated and excepted into WestPoint but at the last minute chickened out and decided not to go, surprised the Dr. was able to ascertain this information with yes and no questions at least now he was listening. The shoulder problem developed because of unresolved emotions relating to this decision. Sounds reasonable the therapist thought so now what?

The chiropractor went on with the testing to ascertain if this was the incident that caused the issue and both were surprised to find in the testing it was not.

"Did the incident originate five years earlier? No!"

"Six years? No!"

"Seven years? No!"

"Eight years, Yes!"

What happened eight years before you went off to college that had anything at all with your decision about attending military school? That would have put the therapist about ten years old?

Then suddenly, as if a light bulb went on he remembered when he was ten he was over at his friend, who suddenly started crying because of his own recently married mother and new stepfather decided to send the friend at the start of the new school year to military school. And he was scared to death!

The chiropractor said your experience when you were ten influenced your decision to go to WestPoint when you graduated high school and you have repressed this ever since. He stood behind the therapist put his hand on the sore spot and snapped his fingers as he said in a firm voice "I release that emotion!"

The therapist walked out a bit perplexed at the whole incident, more bewildered at the fact that the kinetic test could unveil such hidden memories, but more than that within the next day the shoulder completely cleared up and never returned. After a month the therapist even went back to the orthopedic surgeon friend and had another X-ray taken that just showed the gap in the shoulder completely tightened back up, something thought completely medically impossible. When the surgeon asked; "What did you do?" The therapist could only say; "Nothing, absolutely nothing!"

The shoulder is the most mobile joint in the body with its ability to go in almost any direction, and the fact that it was the right arm effect, decisions of what is right in a particular life of this young man might actually play a role in the area of affliction?

This story is absolutely true because I am or was the therapist at the time!

Peter Colla

Truth Hidden In the Dollar

Investigators will tell you, that if you want to find the truth and expose the criminal, look at those who are doing the most talking, you will often find them telling the lies, and since lies are not based on actual events, they will inevitably give away the light as they describe the shadow in their darkness.

We are taught that our bodies are everything. The Physicality of where we are right now, exactly how we feel right this moment is pretty much the major aspect of any disease or problem we might face physically.

The essence of any injury can be analyzed and then if the structures that are injured or affected could somehow be reversed the issue or disease should disappear as well. Nice thought, makes sense and it pretty much takes the thinking out of any problem. The tumor appears, remove the tumor, problem gone?

Unfortunately as is the case in most issues the problem doesn't seem to disappear but merely reappears later in another spot.

Mind Over Matter, the Power of Positive Thinking, Law of Attraction, The Placebo Effect, or various other areas of ideology that put power in the mere way we think, have begun to spring up in various areas of the treatment environment, yet it only seems to get the most fringed recognition, often being spouted as a sort of heresy, how dare we think we can tell the doctors anything, they know it all?

Belief? Well, forget that the spirit, that's pretty much for the miracle department, and those only seem to happen to other people, often fabricated or just some miss-diagnosis that someone else completely fumbled.

Maybe this is more because injuries have a way of defining our lives?

Speak to anyone who has an injury long enough and you will find that for the most place people can speak of nothing else other than the injury they are dealing with, and more so the symptoms.

I have noticed that when people are hurt or dealing with a healthcare issue their whole world becomes this issue, and regardless of how actually small, the issue is. I have known people who have nothing more than a sore pinky toe, and their entire life seems to revolve around this one particular issue. They only think about the toe, they consider the toe, they look at it, they feel it, they see it, they only seem to hear words that speak of it, their whole life revolves around it as if it is some sort of dark black hole, and they have suddenly become trapped in its ever constricting and crushing orbit, spinning down deeper and deeper until death itself seems to become a Mercy?

The injury through fear and deceit causes your eyes, ears, and every thought to dwell on the issue at hand.

It does seem like a self-defeating and self-demeaning manner, to be an almost worship-like consideration of the little toe, two words commonly associated with people becoming patients. Self-Defeating, just look at the word; we defeat ourselves. The other Self-Demeaning; we De-Meaning ourselves or reduce the actual meaning of ourselves as people. That pretty much sums up what happens in the process.

People have a tendency to turn their faces to the ground, they press their faces into the muck and their whole world becomes consumed with the injury. They become a slave to the injury, regardless of how insignificant it is in proportion to the whole body, the effect on the family, or its resulting waves throughout the entire community.

But let us get back to the symbol of people as we are taught.

If we would consider the perspectives of this taught view of us, we might see ourselves maybe like a pyramid, let us take the one off the one-dollar bill as an example;

Our life represented by the monolithic representation of the pyramid, as is so demonstrated throughout history. Pharaohs, leaders all around the world have used this pyramid structure as a representation or demonstration of the life these many great people, countries, cultures have presented, as a way to represent, to "Re-Present" it to us.

So let's take the representation of the pyramid; in this model, the body is the huge base covering the mass that rests against the earth, grounded and needing at least the majority of our consideration for anything to continue, unmovable and face down in the dirt?

The mind then would be the middle section, less than the body but sitting above directing the whole comings and goings of the body, visible and aware of its place in the whole picture; above the body, kind of like the mind or head resting on top of the body, the director, the boss?

Well, then what is the spirit? That little all-seeing eye that kind of floats above, small, insignificant, detached, it radiates with some kind of detached power, floating above, staring out into space or whatever, and just hovers there not really doing anything at all, inconsequential?

If they lie about one thing then are they lying about everything?

Well, what if the opposite is true?

A sort of reverse pyramid image might appear, where the point is down and it expands upward?

What if the body is actually the very smallest portion of the whole? The physical body being the smallest portion of your soul. The very tip but a fraction actually touching the surface of the world? The soul is in essence then the entire aspect of your life in this physical life and beyond, the whole pyramid. The sharpest and insignificant point actually touches the ground, this is in the reality of this moment. The body expands upward and outward for about one-third of the evident structure, blending into the mind the realized experienced life, going up into the clouds infinite and comprising belief. Now, this might make sense?

Science would tell us that the body is merely a conglomeration of assembled atoms, coordinated in the most complex fashion, so perfectly constructed they can hardly understand it let alone fathom it, yet they are convinced, and it is commonly taught, that all atoms are merely various organized structurally restricted entities of energy, locked in particular structures and orbits around each other. Further, these structures are organized into complex patterns and infinitely arranged yet orderly combinations that somehow make us up as humans, this goes for the most part, the entire visible and invisible universe? Reality is now and only present for just this one particular moment in time.

The mind lets assume, in turn, rests above larger and growing upward structures expanding, it might make sense seeing how the mind not only encompasses everything in the now, taking all of its stimulus from every aspect the body might offer but also incorporating these into memory; past, present, and even to a degree that which we might imagine a future, in addition to all this it also extrapolates this information making judgments as to the effects of the past on present information and a possible projection into a theoretical future predictions based on data received to date. A sort of enormous library with shelves for past experiences, interpretation, and reactions to be placed for future reference and deductions.

Then what about the spirit? If it rests above and is the essence of our belief system, being how we believe, it might make sense that it is a product of everything that the mind processes, all the stimulations the body feels at any one particular time, fed up into the mind, processed along with dreams, teachings, imagination given to us through conscience and even un-conscience stimulus, and then passed on to the belief system, "the Spirit" to assemble and collect, building its own collection of experiences as it was to make its own ultimate decision; what does the person actually believe? Does it swing toward yes or no, good or bad, dark or light, God or something else?

If this be the case and the spirit resides up and into heavenly realms of considerations, one might also assume in our structural demonstration that the spirit would go on and upward actually without an end?

So back to health care;

If we are actually structures of not only physicality in the present, but also past, present and to a degree future, and more importantly the mind has a much greater volume of consideration of the whole, than the body, then one would and must assume that the spirit has the greatest consideration if for no other reason then the massive volume of the whole it seems to be in charge of the above structures.

The first step in confronting and eventually eliminating any medical issue a person may be suffering from on an ongoing basis starts with a simple but necessary first step; it is first necessary to understand the issue at hand and exactly what we are fighting.

If we walk into a room and suddenly it smells a little like smoke, even the smallest fraction, a good firefighter would recognize this possibly as a bare wire or some other issue that could possibly be sparking or precipitating flame. If he or she looks at the flame and immediately knows to douse it with water, or correct it with an adjustment in use, the flame goes out and a larger issue is extinguished. A small mess might have to be cleaned, but utter destruction is avoided. It is in this way people of faith can treat leapers and not contract the issue themselves.

Given the fact that we are the greatest proportion of our essence is spirit then we must also realize that anything that happens to us good or bad in our lives is primarily spirit-based, and knowing this makes it so much easier to fight and defeat in the case of a negative confrontation.

We have been taught we have little or no influence on the outcomes or issues that afflict us, that we ourselves are some sort of random occurrences in the infinite vastness of the universe, and when bad things happen to us it is just Karma, bad luck, or being at the wrong place at the wrong time. This is a lie! This misconception has the effect of taking the Divine out of our paths, our very souls, and makes us a bit of a slave to whatever infirmity that may present itself. It is so easy with such thought to just give up and not even begin to hope when we are suddenly afflicted with some sort of dreadful occurrence.

We are taught that the actual specifics of the injuries are too complex to understand and must be left to the people who have actually been taught these facts. As a matter of fact, we are systematically being taught we should not even question the diagnosis or prognosis when told to us, merely act on the results, and do what we are being told.

Ultimately we have been enslaved by the fear of the vast and apparently invincible nature of sicknesses, a false deception regarding their complexity, and false teaching regarding the limits of what we can do about them, or to whom we may look for help. Yet the truths of revealed lies, like having the lights being turned on at night, open our eyes to an obstacle when realized lying in the path on the way to the bathroom, it helps us not stumble and step over the issue as easy as a misplaced thumbtack. These obstacles then demonstrate themselves merely as they truly are; something small, a nuisance, and something you merely have to step over.

"When you lift your head up, start to ask for wisdom, God is faithful to give all you will need to overcome any issue you may seek help with."

Raccoons and Spies

The Raccoon story is a great example I have received as to how people let sicknesses in themselves and they usually suffer the consequences afterward unaware an attack has even happened.

What do sicknesses possibly have to do with Raccoons?

The first step in confronting and eventually eliminating any medical issue a person may be suffering from on an ongoing basis it is first necessary to understand the issue at hand and exactly what we are fighting.

Given the fact that we are in the greatest proportion of our essence spirit, then we must also realize that anything that happens to us, good or bad in our lives, is primarily spirit-based, and knowing this, makes it so much easier to fight and defeat in each specific case the negative confrontation.

As I already said; we have been taught we have little or no influence on the outcomes of issues that afflict us, that we are some sort of random occurrence and when bad things happen to us it is just Karma, bad luck, or being at the wrong place at the wrong time. This misconception has the effect of taking the Divine out of our paths and makes us a bit of a slave to whatever infirmity that may present itself. Thus, making us become prey to the attack, it is so easy with such thought to just give up and not even begin to hope when we are suddenly afflicted with a dreadful occurrence.

If we will further suppose that all injuries of any type are attacks, then like any type of attack, there is a specific direction from which it comes, there is a weakness in our own personal defenses that this attack and others like it may have breached, and if we can identify exactly what direction and in what manner the attack is occurring, we can use this information to fight back!

You can only effectively fight an attacking hoard if you are facing them when they attack. In war, information is key to victory.

I can remember with not such fond recollection living up in the forest and deciding one day to take the kids on a picnic for the evening. We made a whole bunch of baked chicken, packed up all the supplies, and headed off to the lake many miles away.

What I didn't realize was we left one of the containers of the chicken out on the counter cooling. There were a few, so missing one was not noticeable. Neither did the boys notice the window they left open earlier that day. We didn't notice anything until we got home late that night and saw that the house had been ransacked, the cushions were destroyed, everything had been toppled over, and the place looked and smelled like a garbage bomb went off! We had been living in this home, in the forest for years, and never had such an attack before. Amazing what a couple of little raccoons could do.

"So what do we know about Raccoons?"

Anyone who might on an occasion or two had the privilege of running into a close encounter with raccoons might have a story quite similar to this one.

This particular raccoon story manifested as it were in the home that I enjoyed out in the middle of the forest, unaware and ill-prepared for the mess that was about to come.

One summer weekend we decided to spend the afternoon at the lake, going through the usual preparations, buying and packing all the necessary food and entertainment materials we would need for the day.

The kids would pack the things they might need or use, and we would prepare the food in advance, making it easier to just have fun and not have to worry about bringing all the cooking supplies a longer and more complex dinner preparation might require. In this particular trip, Chicken was on the menu, three trays to be exact, all of which were prepared grilled to cooked perfection beforehand.

The chicken, three trays cooled on the counter, for we were having all of the extended family join us as well, and the baskets were filled and packed for the lunch and evening feast. All the materials were placed in the various picnic baskets we brought, and as soon as the truck was loaded we were off.

It wasn't until the evening dinner that we realized that we had left one of the three trays of chicken behind. Not a devastating problem for we had prepared extra and had plenty of the other food to feed everyone. Campfire and the customary evening fun, pack up a bit later and went home.

As we opened the door of the home we realized the place was in shambles, mess everywhere, couches were torn up, garbage, chicken bones and stink all over the floors. The mess, damage, and feces were everywhere, and suddenly I heard a sound coming from the boy's bedroom. We quickly turned on the light and grabbed a broomstick heading cautiously down the hall towards the room for we still weren't sure what we were dealing with, a "bear" becomes a real possibility at least until we actually laid eyes on it.

But unfortunately, or perhaps, fortunately, the creatures escaped out of the window in the boy's room. There were clearly dirty animal tracks up the wall and out the open window; Raccoons!

My son was wide-eyed, and a bit scares as he realized he had left the window open that morning. He left the window open, I left the bait in the form of the chicken, the raccoons decided to show up and have a party.

"The raccoon attack is as sicknesses, the mess is what happens when it stays awhile unnoticed."

Therapy briefly, yet to be discussed more in-depth later; now the first thing we did was turn on the light! Yes, that had the effect of scaring away the animals, maybe they just heard our talking, but most likely they wanted to just get away seemingly undetected since they were obviously full having accomplished what they came for; chicken dinner!

But low and behold the damage was done, the house was in

shambles and some of the destruction may not even be able to be repaired depending on the extent of the damage done.

"This storm and the winds of menacing raccoons is a perfect example of sicknesses and the effects they have on the body."

The next step was to close the window! If we had not realized that animals were even there and merely assumed maybe the house was burglarized or even more absurd; an earthquake or a tornado inside the house may have done this, one may have not made the connection between the window and the attack. Once the after cleanup efforts were complete and everyone went to bed, the now newly hungered raccoons may have returned to perform another examination of the refrigerator or perhaps the trash this time.

Silly how if people never realize they have a raccoon infestation, or a problem leaving windows open and food out on the counter, one might begin to think they are just unlucky or have a bad house, prone to strange and sudden spontaneous garbage explosions from out of the garbage bin. Opening the mind to all the possibilities of the mess allows us to realize the true culprits and secure the situation so the event doesn't repeat itself.

But if our pioneers of the rugged forest are clever enough to realize they not only left the window open but may have even baited the animals in, closing off these two factors quickly reduces the chances for reoccurrence and leaves them with step three of the true rehabilitation; "mopping up the mess."

People sit and take it, thinking the mess or the bruises are the sicknesses, while the actual malevolent attack has long gone, or worse they sit in their house unaware of the continuing inflicting damage the returning raccoons do.

So like the raccoons we must identify the issues and then look for them, turn on the lights, maybe get loud, and they will just run off?

Yes, like the raccoons in the story the first moment you become aware an attack has occurred or you are in the process of an attack you must turn on the Light, then do something that basically prompts it to leave.

God is the Light!

But if not a raccoon perhaps the image of a spy might also work when describing the processes around diseases or afflictions. As in war, or peace, spies will infiltrate into societies, organizations, or systems, even computer systems, mimicking entities that seem normal or legitimate, but inside their motivations are of malice instead of health, motives of destruction instead of growth.

As in war and peace, a spy can infiltrate a social circle and through the infliction of damage or theft, can place a balanced and successful social structure suddenly in turmoil. But let us not forget the spy is not a friend, he is an entity that wishes to illicit malice. From the outside and with the wrong information, people might believe as the structures or functions suddenly begin to dissimilate the problem merely lies in a spontaneous breakdown of normal functions common with a complex working structure. When subsequent repairs are performed and the same structures or other related ones suddenly follow the perplexing result is a sort of cat chasing its own tail scenario develops whereby people may throw water on a fire but if a person doesn't address the fire starter, the nasty little brat with the box of matches, more fires will just irrupt later.

The good news is as in the case of the spy, merely realizing that there may be an outside agent or spy, inflicting these attacks, will have the profound result of putting the fear of God into it. Thus, chasing first the spy off, and then when subsequent repairs occur, there is no repeated destruction or continual disruption occurring.

Spy's, like cockroaches, know when they are being hunted, they are the most basic of creatures, and while they may be cunning they are also cowards and have no stomach for direct confrontation, regardless of how many James Bond movies may speak to the contrary.

So what exactly happens when we suddenly put the light on and the cockroach is spotted, he runs like crazy. Sickness is every bit the same.

Look to God first, light is turned on, and then the answers will be given.

Most people, especially those who are suffering, "have not because they ask not."

So let us for a moment assume we did ask, and the light turned on, what next? After this initial turning on of the light, realizing we are under attack and it's just not something we have suddenly become, we must pick up the weapons we have been given, this just makes our task easier, to realize the next possible task and that there is the need to drive them out.

It is amazing but when you look at the healing Jesus

demonstrated and see them not only through the body, mind, and spiritual perspective but also from a health care practitioner, it is clear He gave us so many examples of this. As a matter of fact, He gave us a complete and thorough program of how you should rid yourselves of all these afflictions.

The Spirit of God brought all the necessary specific examples to his followers so they could write them down, in a way that completely documents everything each of us needs to free ourselves of any and all afflictions.

It is believed that Jesus healed millions of people, in the short span of His actual teaching life, as a matter of fact, he healed in one way or another every single person He came in contact with. For it was written, *"if they had written down every miracle He had performed it would fill all the books ever written in the world."*

I didn't need to bombard you the reader with endless repetition of miracle after miracle, only speak of the significant ones that describe how not only you must identify God in everything around you, but see the spiritual side of sicknesses if you truly want to combat them thoroughly and effectively from every perspective you are afflicted.

Belief

If you are going to experience healing to its fullest or even embrace the healing God has promised you then a good first step is the stepping stone of Belief? You must be willing to believe, or at the very least accept the notion that it may be true.

"Belief is the greatest portion of life, it is the greatest portion of healing."

I must say that with the majority of people I have treated throughout my career, the belief at least revolving around the prospect of success with healing is a product largely dependent on the person's own personal belief. This too has changed over the course of the last thirty years, people through the media or educational institutions that supply the internet draw their own conclusions about the prognosis of the injury they are suffering from based on these statements they read or hear, usually drawing their own conclusions long before they enter the office of a care provider.

Having this information, while many would think is good, also when it speaks doubt into their lives gives them increased hopelessness because if they happen to read there is nothing that can be done for a particular ailment, regardless of what someone of faith or positive belief might say, they already have become convinced of the outcome regarding what they believe is the truth.

A person has to believe or at least be willing to start to think they can be healed, or perhaps deserve to be healed, to actually have the ability to see healing they may already have received? How many people come in with the predisposed idea that they are receiving exactly what they "deserve" either by actions by themselves or even just by the heritage of their birth?

I would say the answer to this question is; the majority, all if I had to be honest, every single person I had ever treated where the subject actually came up when they actually took responsibility, (that is with the exception of children), usually had what they felt was a predisposed origin for the affliction they were suffering. They all uniformly believed they were suffering as a result of their own path or actions, and in almost every case felt that is why they remained ill. While others would heal, or escape the persecution these sicknesses seemed to cause, they would in most cases say approximately the same thing; "I did it to myself, I did this or that, played this or that sport, partied too much, walked down this or that path I knew I shouldn't, and that is why I have this today, and why others get better and I don't. You have no idea what I have done!"

To a degree they are right, the majority of afflictions could be avoided by the choice of specific paths in life or not, but the idea of whether or not one deserves healing falls right in line with the concept of deserving forgiveness or not. This right is the gift granted to each and every person through the death of God's Son, and thus a free gift to all who are willing to accept it.

People, for the most part, seem to be willing to ask for forgiveness for things, especially when they clearly know they are doing wrong at the moment and chose this particular direction anyway. They will also forgive others, especially if they are good in their hearts, even enemies or people who have done horribly wrongs towards them, but where people, in general, have the greatest amount of issue is forgiving themselves, this holds back healing often more than anything else? They speak with their thoughts and prayers; "Lord please heal my diabetes," which is no different than; remove me from this storm I am suffering from as I continue to go down this road towards what I know is dark clouds, or at least claim it upon myself with my own words.

If you listen very closely to what is being said; "Lord Heal" and then "My Diabetes" on one hand they want to overcome it and on the other they claim it!

You can't have both, and as children who are created in the image of God; your words have power, it was written in God's Word; That you will be accountable for your every word, a Promise, and a truth.

"Now let me tell you what I know about Michelle?"

Michelle

I love to use as the example of the power of believing the story of my wife Anna's friend Michelle. Michelle personally gave Anna permission to use her name and example when helping other people, so I will use her real name.

Michelle was a client of Anna during the time she was teaching Pilates in Amsterdam and was a loyal attendant of the class for many years, and as many such friendships develop they became more friends than just instructor and client. After a great deal of time, Michelle came in one day and said to Anna; "I will not be coming into Pilates anymore."

When Anna pressed her to find out why Michelle finally broke down and shared with her that she had been struggling with bone and blood cancer for years, and recently she had seen the doctor and heard it had returned stage 4. She would have to start soon the most aggressive form of chemotherapy at least twenty treatments in six months, and it would probably leave her completely incapacitated.

to

The most difficult question was asked; "What are your chances?" The doctors said with the chemo, she had six months, without it, it could be only weeks?

After much crying, as many a friend would do, the question was posed; "Have you tried absolutely everything?"

And while Michelle assured her she had, yet she was willing to look once again in any possible alternative. Calling all of her friends and searching endless hours in alternative healing options there in Holland and abroad, they finally came across one spiritual healer they had until then not heard of. A spiritual healer in Brazil claiming to examine the patient and then pray and whatever God tells him to have the patient do, they are instructed to do.

So they thought what can it hurt let's call him. At first, the healer stated they would have to come in front of him for the process to work, but for Michelle, the thought of traveling all the way to Brazil was too much, so they thanked the healer but couldn't come. He felt pity for the two women and said; "I never do this but go ahead and send me your picture, and I will try to pray while looking at it and see if God says anything to me?"

After receiving the picture he called them back and said to

the two women "this is what I was told when I prayed; put on a pure white gown and lie down in bed, pray to God to open your eyes, and whoever you see, whatever they have done, pray to God to forgive them, even if with only words. And this is the most important part; forgive yourself for your part in this problem." "I hope this helps, God bless." He hung up.

The two women were a little disappointed, hoping perhaps the healer would give them healing and not just advice, but they went out and bought the white clothes anyway, and while they didn't lie down on the bed they did go to the ocean and scream out loud, crying and praying. Michelle was Vietnamese one of the Boat-People from the late sixties early seventies, coming to America with her mother. While she remembered scattered memories of her past, she really had little or no memories of her time before coming to America even though she was nearly eleven when she arrived. But suddenly as these prayers rang out she suddenly started having vivid and complete memories of her childhood she had locked away so many years earlier, the time while living in Vietnam.

She suddenly began to remember being systematically and repeatedly raped by her father and uncle, and many of his friends for years, all the way back to being a very little child. What made things worse, is that she also remembered that when she tried to tell her mother, she was immediately and repeatedly silenced as to not bring shame upon their family.

It was commonly known by many people that Michelle had her whole life been ashamed of being Vietnamese, but it wasn't until this moment did she understood why she always hated her blood, and even her heritage, her very bones!

They quickly remembered the instruction of the Brazilian Healer to forgive whoever came to mind even if it is with words only, as difficult as it was; "Mouth the words out loud if nothing else." This whole process seemed to take all afternoon as the faces of all the assailants began to rush across her memory and each needing in their turn to be forgiven one after another.

They finally finished at the sea and went back to Anna's apartment where Michelle was so exhausted from the ordeal she just wanted to lay down. As all the memories flooding in finally brought her up to the age and point where she had active adult memories, and consequentially all the forgiveness words were spoken, Anna reminded her "now you have to also forgive yourself," perhaps the hardest thing one can be asked to do.

Michelle spoke out the words of forgiveness of herself for

hating her own life, her blood, her heritage, her very bones, and forgave herself for her self-hatred. At the very moment she just spoke those final words through the tears and sobs, she suddenly fell back in the bed asleep, seemingly completely exhausted from the work.

After the second day straight of Michelle not waking up Anna began to be concerned, checking up with her, but she seemed to be sleeping soundly and decided not to wake her. After nearly three days of non-stop sleep suddenly she woke up, she looked better and more rested than she had appeared the entire time Anna knew her. As a matter of fact, she stated she had never felt better.

The first chemo appointment was scheduled for the following Friday, and as was customary she had to go in for tests to make sure the dosage was correct. Upon completing the first test the doctor was baffled by the result; it showed absolutely no trace of cancer in her blood. It was so low, basically zero, he wondered if his own test had been broken or faulty so much so that he ordered the test taken two more times at two different labs all with the same result.

The Cancer had vanished! Not only had it vanished but she had absolutely not a single trace of any cancer whatsoever in her body. This fact also was perplexing to the doctor because everyone usually has at least a trace of these cells being tested for, but Michelle didn't have any.

I would like to say this story had a happy ending, but the doctors not believing even the results of their own test still forced Michelle with the threat of cancelation of her insurance to continue the chemo regiment anyway, stating that perhaps the cancer is merely hidden?

A few months later Michelle died of complications from pneumonia she developed while on the chemo.

As you can see the single most powerful weapon on the planet in the spiritual realm is forgiveness, and forgiving yourself is absolutely essential for any assurance of the healing process will be manifested and more importantly completed, of this point, we will discuss later.

Why did Michelle die if she was healed? Some would say, the same factors should have been effective that cured the initial cause of her issue, would they not cure the symptoms affecting her body? But like the fire, while the water might put out the early flame, it doesn't reverse the burning and char caused by time-related damage. So like a person who just put out a flame, immediately bringing inflammable materials into our house especially when embers are still fresh, weaknesses in the structure, a new and possible different fire, and the person runs the risk of another ignition of symptoms?

If the healing and forgiveness closed the window or door in her house, fear opened it back up; the fear of always needing to go back and re-check, run another test, take another precautionary dose of medication ultimate placing in herself combustibles that when the attack came initiated again this time she was too weak to fight back. If forgiveness closes the doors to our castle fear certainly can open them up again. Her life may have been much more of an inspiration being able to tell such her story herself, but her story, her victory even in facing death, in the memories of everyone who knew her and saw the miracles that occurred know the truth and will never forget.

She did tell it herself and is an inspiration of the truth, this is the true definition of a Martyr's death.

While Michelle knew where the mess was in her life, she never examined the actual causes until right before the end. She still died.

Perhaps on a spiritual level, her purpose had been fulfilled, to teach Anna and through her, you the significance of

Forgiveness in the healing process. Forgiveness is one of the most powerful weapons of cleansing in the life you have been given.

Why some people die and others don't, specifically why did Michelle have to die then, for the same reason my first wife and child died when they did because it was their time. And as any doctor who is actually honest about the fact of life and death as it relates to health care and treatments of today, will tell you that ultimately the decision of who lives and dies has nothing to do with the doctor and everything to do with God, at least this is a fact by one who admits believing in God might?

There is also a dark side to medicine that is so evil, some of these ghoul-like vultures once some of them get their talons into somebody they will not let go unless they are absolutely made to. I have known many friends and patients who have been given life-threatening treatments or expensive procedures they didn't even need, such as chemotherapy either before any diagnosis of cancer was confirmed or even for other issues, where these chemicals normally would not be prescribed. Such so-called cutting-edge treatments cost tens of thousands of dollars each and the doctors can make hundreds of thousands of dollars on a single patient.

On a spiritual level these destructive and aggressive so-called treatments, which by the way are not a "treat" but a "trick", a "trick or treat", actually place the person's life at risk, for one purpose only, and that is to weaken them and systematically drain every resource from them and their families until the person is left with a dried up skeleton-like body that mimics death, so much so, that when the person being attacked looks in the mirror they lose all desire for life and actually want death.

In the case of Michelle and others that find themselves in the clutches of these medical ghouls, it is clear with the dark shadow in the eyes of the person coercing these innocents into the gas chambers of death, or the evil smirk of unrelated greed and power that demonstrates a clear attitude that has nothing to do with healing or even interest in the wellbeing of the person standing before them but has an absolute desire to control and inflict their desires of destruction regardless of the wants and desire of the person or the loved ones around them.

When medical procedures, pills, or advice cause so much pain, misery, or what appear to be a direct and aggressive turn away from everything that is good, godly, or life-giving, there is no way it can be considered Godly, and if it isn't Godly then that only leaves one other thing; darkness.

All I know if our Father loves His children as much as I love my own, then there will be a reckoning for the lustful desire of death issued out upon the innocents for greed!

Reverse Our Thinking

So what do we do about it?

We must reverse our thinking from the perspective of health care. First, we must take our trust away from whom the world has said we must place it, take our eyes off the ground and look to the tree branch as a path to the sky.

We must, if we want to guarantee improvement, as it were, inject good into ourselves in any way possible, with the most complete and encompassing manner, that basically means we must engulf ourselves in goodness, truth, and only the purest Godly sensations through the doors we receive the various stimulus. If Godly goodness baths us through our eyes, ears, through our food, air, water, and basically surrounds our very bodies we leave no gate for darkness to get in.

Doctors, we have been told are in charge of our health care, but are they really? Over the course of the last twenty years, there has been a significant shift in whom is really in charge of our healthcare system especially as related to individuals. As a health care provider, I have seen an increasing shift in control of the care of patients, regarding specifically what could be done for all sorts of medical issues, or more significantly what was acceptable as the approved procedure.

It was a subtle taking over of the authority of health, starting first with all the major providers becoming associated members or Contractees of healthcare insurance carriers. Suddenly approval was required (as stated) to verify that patients were actually covered by insurance carriers. This verification later became mandated, and finally needed in the form of pre-authorization approval to even see the patient, at which time the insurance companies would gradually decide what care, duration, medicine, even specific medicine brand, location, sometimes the specific doctors that may be used, any and all specifics regarding the treatment of any health care issue every individual might need or receive. The insurance companies even went so far as to buy up the majority of the hospitals and many of the medical providers so that they were, in fact, paying themselves, controlling even profiting from every possible aspect of the health care environment. They started actually advising their providers, educating them, and telling the doctors exactly what to say to the patients. If the providers decided to go against the new controls and orders, they were either barred from receiving the authorization for the care they did want to provide or in some cases faced ostracizing from the health care community completely.

So when they tell us, providers, that the only way to treat a specific illness is with this one particular avenue of treatment, to question this option would require the patient to often step completely outside the health care model as a whole, usually risking themselves denials of insurance benefits for care. This presented quite a conundrum for people who instinctively knew that what they were being advised to do for a particular issue was or felt wrong.

I wonder if it is fear, the real unknown, the horrible big bad Boogy-man, we know nothing about, can't see or sense, yet must constantly look over our shoulder for, run another test for, take another vitamin for, that giant invisible thing that keeps people in line when it comes to health care. Maybe it is the control, control of our minds, control of our belief, where or whom we place our trust in, who we have assurance in so we can regain our health when we stumble or fall? Is this the ultimate desire of those who seem to wish to control others?

Reverse our thinking!

Opening our minds to a possibility that if someone or some entity is trying ultimately to control us, more so than trying to help us heal, then we can assume, by such actions against us, that the opposite is true; take our trust off the ground and lift it up to the sky. Time to take our lives back, take back the control of our healthcare. Insurance companies that benefit from the restrictions or denial of care should never be allowed to play a role in the decision-making process, it is a violation of the very regulations that denied doctors the rights to own offices they might benefit from in their patient care recommendations. But here again, we know who writes the laws, big business does we the people certainly do not?

We may not be able to change the system, but we can make a change in our own lives? We must look to our belief system as not only the greatest influence on our lives, but as a possible majority of the reason for any and all issues that we come across, regarding our own healthcare issues, and then consequently the major consideration factor for not only treatment but the actual definition of what is considered true healing.

The True Enemy is Fear

If the dark goal is to create a system of medicine or medical treatments to control people then the controlling agents must first remove all knowledge of the workings of sicknesses by making them so sophisticated that the laymen cannot fathom it, and then place it out of the hands of everyday people, making these solutions unobtainable, without coming to them first for the solution.

Inject a portion of fear, first by making the treatments so expensive that the thought of Insurance or "Assurance" of payment is so ridiculously high that total ruination would follow if one had to pay themselves. And second, by placing fear into the media of the sicknesses themselves, whereby the mere mention of their names like Ebola, stroke, addiction, cancer, autism, manic depression conjures up such images of fright to cause all the masses to cowl in absolute horror? Fear seems to be the goal.

Jesus Himself said; "Fear not" or "Do not fear" more than any other single statement in his ministry.

In my younger days, I have hunted in the western United

States, where its vast spaces and diverse variety of wildlife made for various levels of a challenge even for the most experienced hunters. One fact was commonly known among the most experienced hunters, the difference between being the hunter and being hunted often had to do with levels of confidence or fear.

Wild dogs, for example, are a perfect example of the power of fear. These animals sense fear, and in the wild when they come across other creatures or people for that matter, they will run unless they sense fear, then they suddenly attack! Fear draws in the attackers like flies to sugar!

Fear attracts attacks, and if sicknesses are as an attack, and let us suppose for a moment they may be spirits, then logically fear attracts sicknesses! Dark spirits feed on fear, sicknesses are dark.

In my earlier years, growing up in the Western United States, I had many opportunities to camp, hike, and even on occasion hunt in very remote places where a person might find themselves utterly alone for perhaps miles. On one occasion I had a chance to speak to a very experienced outdoorsman named DJ about mountain lions that frequented the area we were hiking.

Mountain lions are extremely stealthy, and rarely let themselves be seen during the day, and most certainly by people. DJ assured me if you ever see a mountain lion it is probably because he is hunting you.

On this particular trip, I went off and decided to hike down into a small canyon along a game trail just mainly to see the not tree-filled basin and the gentle creek that flowed through the bottom of the canyon. When I got all the way down, I was amazed at the natural beauty of everything around almost like a Garden of Eden look. The surroundings had clear evidence that animals frequented it quite often, there were the obvious signs of depressions in the grass that I assumed were from deer or elk, either way very peaceful and beautiful.

Suddenly I realized in a moment, that I was a long way away from any other persons, my comrade was sleeping back at camp and had no idea where I was, or even which direction I had wandered off to. If I had gotten hurt, or snake-bitten, or anything there was at least tens of square miles of the thick countryside where clearly no human hardly walked. Plus I realized suddenly all I had with me to defend myself was a simple pocket knife, and with the exception of the binoculars I carried, I didn't even carry a canteen with me, and that after the talk of mountain lion only earlier the same day seemed to put a real scare into my mind.

For a moment a touch of fear caressed the back of my neck. Then suddenly I heard a loud snap coming from up the game trail path where I just came down. I might as well have had a bear reach out from the bush and grab my ankle the chill was so strong and even stronger was the sharp distinct concentrated identification of the fearful sound coming from up the path? I stepped behind the nearest tree and tried to look up the path with the binoculars but could only see a large dark brown shape descending along the path halfway up the cliff or higher. The creature looked too big to be a mountain lion, too short to be an elk, but clearly let out at least two or more grunts low and ominous as it broke more sticks and branches as it descended. It was still far up the slope yet the sounds were so magnified by my fear the sound could have been right next to me?

Very rapidly three thoughts went through my head; stay and see what it was as it came closer down the path, yell and make loud noises to possibly scare it away, or rapidly retreat up the canyon and exit out further upstream back to camp. Not knowing for sure what exactly was coming, my mind went immediately to "Bear" and I was not feeling like taking my chances armed only with a pocket knife, so I quickly retreated up the canyon until I found another game trail up and out of the canyon.

The feeling of fear did not leave me until I actually reached the crest of the canyon, and looking back realized nothing was following me.

I later told DJ about the incident and he said to me; "The difference between you and them is you are out there for your fun, for them, it is life and death!" "The difference between being hunter or prey rests only in one thing; your attitude!" "Those creatures and trust me they are animals can sense fear, and like a dog to a bone, they are attracted to it!"

Injuries and sicknesses work the same way!

It has been my experience as a health care provider that people often and almost without exception attract the very sicknesses they fear, especially when they speak of them over and over again with their words, conversations, tests, worries, or even fixations of their minds. Sicknesses are attracted to those who fear them and likewise, when we don't fear them we actually scare them off.

Choose not to fear, it is a choice!

Fear is the greatest cause of dilapidation in human existence.

It is quite clear and now commonly known that people can even die from fear.

The mind has an enormous influence on the body, and when the mind gets overwhelmed with pain signals it is completely possible for a person to die without any clear physical termination of function. Prior to the development of modern anesthetic, people would often die before the operation or procedures could progress even to the point of being life-threatening themselves merely because a person was experiencing such severe pain.

But belief, or what people think they know is true, influences strongly the mind and the interpretation of not only the sensations we feel but what they mean to our well-being, especially when it comes to the future and prospects of fulfilling the dreams of yesterday. Patients will often come in with a predisposed idea of how a process will unfold actually looking for manifested symptoms that qualify those outlooks even before they actually show up. Basically, they believe themselves into becoming sick.

They bathe themselves in negative words of "I have this or that," "I Am susceptible to this or that," "it is in my genes" or even worse start calling themselves this or that sickness survivor, labeling themselves with a blanket of sound and belief in the very thing that they either conquered or fear.

These ideas or ideologies about expected symptoms will often also cause them to become fixated on the issues at hand disregarding everything else revolving around them. This mindset, in essence, concentrates their attention on the smallest structures in their body placing an almost giant-like image on the smallest structure in and on their body, but also, more destructively; placing them into a posture of submission to this smallest irritant and allow it to completely take over their lives. They fear pain and the afflictions of what might happen to them.

People could say pain is "the Enemy's" greatest weapon?

Pain is not of the enemy, pain is the warning system God has built into His children to give us warning of an attack, from what direction, and exactly what is being attacked, even what door or window the attack is trying to use, what path it is trying to impair.

The problem is people try to ignore the pain alarm, dumb them down with narcotics, or teach themselves to just live with it without ever looking at what exactly the alarm bell is trying to tell them? We need to pay attention to the pain and ask what exactly is it trying to tell us? Focus on the pain, not the fear!

Fear is a different experience than pain and what it does to people, it causes people to focus on what is not, taking our minds off all of the rest of what we already have. Fear is the enemy's and sicknesses' greatest weapon! It places the attention on what might be, could be, or would be, but not what is!

God says; "Fear Not" more than anything else, but never say do not have pain. Pain is information, listen to what it is telling you immediately, and act positively and it will stop. Once the fire alarm is responded to and action is taken, it is no longer needing to ring.

As already stated sicknesses are like spies, they often sneak in almost unobservable ways, just to wreak havoc in their malevolent assignments dwelling in darkness hidden until their presence is actually discovered, it is only then that they are either chased off or captured and destroyed.

Sicknesses may act as spies, but in reality, they are so small and insignificant in their creation, almost like insects, yes maybe like the scorpion, they can only harm us if we let them? I have a lot of experience with scorpions in my life, living in the Southwest and having more than a few in my house, even being stung a time or two. A scorpion is a quiet and for the most part docile little creature, but when it gets agitated it becomes crazy and goes immediately on the attack, yes it will even go into such a frenzy causing often a risk of its own life, for it is in the scorpion's nature to let anger overwhelm it with foolishness. Foolishness allows it to expose itself, give up the ghost as it were and make an easy target for illumination for those who are calm enough to look. A simple boot is usually all it takes to illuminate the threat!

The larger the creature, the harder and more pinpoint the attack plan must be.

Jesus showed even this, in some cases, demons can only be freed from attacking hosts through prayer and fasting. Fasting is one of the greatest tools you can use for activating heavenly reactions to earthly issues. We will get into the advantages and Godly gifts associated with fasting and the enormous health benefits these simple programs can initiate in the body, but for now, we will simply say, sometimes, some issues take a little more action and thought purely because of the complexity of the attacking hoard?

The reality of the spy! As I said earlier in war and even in peace, in sickness or in health, a spy-like spirit can infiltrate a social circle and through the infliction causing damage or theft, can place a balanced and successful social structure suddenly in turmoil. From the outside and with the wrong information, people might believe as these structures or functions suddenly begin to dissimilate the problem merely lies in a spontaneous breakdown of normal function common with any complex working structure. Basically, they look at themselves as faulty rather than even contemplating an attack from the outside?

When subsequent repairs are performed, and the same structures or other related ones suddenly follow in a destructive failure event of a body part or system, the perplexing result is a sort of cat chasing its own tail scenario develops whereby people may throw water on the fire, but if a person doesn't address the fire starter more fires will just irrupt.

The good news is as in the case of the spy or the sickening spirit, merely realizing that there may be an outside agent, a menacing shadow, or spy, inflicting these attacks, will have the profound result of chasing first the spy off and then when subsequent repairs occur there is little or no repeated destruction or continual disruption occurring.

Sicknesses, infirmities, malevolent spirits, like cockroaches, like spies, are among the most basic spirit and animal world, their cunning is primitive at best, but they do know when they are being hunted. They are the most basic of creations, little angry scorpions, and while they may be merciless in their attacks, they are also cowards and never have a stomach for direct confrontation, regardless of what Hollywood or a million drug company adds would tell us to the contrary?

"So what exactly happens when we suddenly put the light on and the sickening cockroach is spotted; he runs like crazy! Sicknesses of all sorts are every bit the same."

You know you are under attack, the first thing you do is turn on the light. Look to God for answers, and ask Him about what tools you should use to fight the issue at hand. Ask God for help scaring away the attacking foe, and ask God what needs to be learned in the process, the "why me" aspects, and finally "the what now" after the attack has vanished.

It is my experience that sicknesses can be classified into these three distinct but useful examples; the Raccoons, the Bully, or the Spy. So when the lights come on and a person realizes they may have an issue with raccoons in the house, we know what is the next step.

Realizing what exactly we are dealing with is the first and only step in overcoming any enemy in any battle. A person cannot enter into any fight whether it be by their own choice or something thrust upon them and hope to have any chance of victory if they go in blind, or Heaven forbid facing the wrong direction. The medical community as we know it would have us deal with issues basically blind, telling us to trust not only the analysis of our health to them, but the contemplation and eventual choice of treatment directions, even as much as to whether we treat at all? All left to the decision-making authorities of people who seemingly know as little about us as individuals as they seem to care.

Time to take charge of the situation! Grab a big stick and commence in the chasing away faze!

Prayer and Forgiveness

Turning on the light, as simple of an act as that is in a house, the mere reaching over and flicking a switch on the wall, can be the simplest act one can do in a dark room where it is clear by the sensations being felt that something is amiss. Turning on the light has an immediate and profound effect, especially on the simplest of creatures. The scattering, running, or fleeing that occurs happens immediately.

I had the misfortune or perhaps now that I realize it, the fortune, early in my career in needing to rent an apartment that was a bit older and perhaps poorer than one I might venture to try today. I can remember on more than one occasion walking into the kitchen in the middle of the night to retrieve a glass of water stepping on something, and realizing by the recognizable crunch that I had stepped on a cockroach. Funny as it was, while the lights were out, it didn't matter how much ruckus I made or even if one or more of their buddies even got stepped on, they merely stayed put.

It wasn't until the lights actually went on, that a massive run for cover frenzy occurred? In the dark, these small creatures were not afraid even in near sure death of my foot, but when the lights came on there was scattering from all directions, going in all directions, running into each other, bouncing off solid objects, a just trying desperately to find any spot where a shadow or darkness might present cover again.

If calling on, or looking up to God, represents an instant turning on of the light, then one could conclude the same effect happens at the very moment the action is facilitated. A simple beginning is a statement such as "God bless" or "God help me" or perhaps more specifically "Go away in the name of God" should be enough to facilitate scattering!

So early on in my attempts to initiate Godly healing into the practicing medical procedures I gave, I tried prayer, and while I never actually prayed out loud to a single one of my patients, I would under my breath pray for them as I worked on them. I even over the course of the following couple of months trying to pray and then seeing if they could actually feel the difference or not.

I never considered myself much of a praying person, my own Christian upbringing seemed to embed into my mind at least a blueprint of how it should actually go, at least I hoped, but not much seems to come out. Most of the time the prayer was more or less me asking for something from God, not completely different from the more than a few times I had prayed throughout my own life. But for the most, the actual prayer amounted to me quietly asking God to bless the person I was working on, heal them or take away their pain. This seeming to be basically all I could seem to muster at the time.

I was amazed to realize that often the patients themselves could actually feel something and on many occasions would ask me "Are you doing something different, because suddenly it feels so much better?" This in itself was perplexing and fascinating. But still, I was wondering often regarding the patients, especially while speaking of an immediate reduction of pain or tension, these reported reductions only lasted hours or moments for that matter, sustaining relief just to have the symptoms return shortly after they left, or sometimes at least until the next day. This amounted to a question, at least in my own mind; "Did the prayer do anything or did it just amount to a sort of placebo effect even in my own treating method?"

Again part of the problem was while I was praying for the person, I was also praying to have the pain taken away, not yet realizing that the pain was trying to tell us something? Praying for the wrong thing basically amounts to throwing the right punches in a fight, except pointed in the wrong direction. How hilarious of a spectacle for spiritual creatures as they sit there and laugh at the bumbling child trying to fight blind.

Yet I also now know that we as people have no idea the power of prayer, next to love it is the most powerful force in the entire universe. I think if we could see in the spiritual what is going on, as related to our words spoke, we would be amazed. In essence, we have no idea the life-giving and life-taking effects our very words have. But God did show me a glimpse back then at least to open my eyes to the reality of prayer, a gift, a grace, so let me show you this glimpse as well.

Sickness is a crisis, and a crisis is a storm, then logically; sickness is a storm.

Being in a place of acceptance even if this is just a spiritual place, and not just the passing social/economical moments of our lives, can and always seems to leave us in a position of vulnerability that pulls at the very strings of our mind and soul. That feeling of uncertainty, accountability, openness, trends us to question our own stability in an already unstable world.

It is no wonder why everyone hates crisis, not to mention the usual resulting manifesting conflicts that always seem to fill us with dread, fear, and a deep feeling of insignificance, makes us stand back and look at ourselves often with resulting realization of how small we really are. This, of course, plays havoc with our self-esteem and/or the lack thereof, making us just cherish every moment we live in crisis (I was being facetious), bringing to mind the scripture "consider yourself glad when you are being persecuted"! This is a very difficult situation and concept to wrap our arms around. How can we possibly count ourselves glad when we are in crisis? The answer; knowing that there is an opportunity for change and through this change, we can become better people.

I am no stranger to crisis, and if anyone knows me they also realize that crisis has been my middle name over the course of the last forty or so years. Thank God for this crisis, for it is through these many crisis situations that God has truly done its work in my life.

In a great line from the movie The Shawshank Redemption, the narrating character remembers a quote from his friend "You can get started living, or you can get on started dying?"

I believe in any true crisis, we find ourselves at one pivotal point where we must choose to "Get busy living, or get busy dying," this choice, whether we want to admit it or not, often manifests itself in the active drawing close to God or a departure from him. Death is what waits for us if we depart from Him!

I'd like to think that I have chosen wisely, and I am drawing closer to Him than away, but at the same time, realizing that He is all around us and in us; it is myself that will somehow on a spiritual level draws closer or move away. Now that presents itself with a difficult dilemma, how do we move away from something that completely and utterly surrounds and comprises every aspect of the world we live in, including us! It would seem that it would be like jumping in a pool and then just by a pure act of will, or choice, decide we don't want to be wet! Or maybe it is concentrating on one small factor of reality and disregarding everything else, like a sore little toe?

I'd like to think I ponder on a regular basis such philosophical thoughts, but to be honest I have a hard time contemplating whether or not I should water the trees in my yard, let alone my place in the universe in reference to God.

It is for this reason that I believe God gives us visions and dreams, if He had to wait around for us meager Humans to ponder a deep thought, especially in this age where we are being bombarded with every aspect of mind-numbing, psycho-distractions, I believe He'd be waiting until He was blue in the face, which He could be right now, who really knows the face of God? My point is; in the muck and mire I call my life at this particular moment, God in his infinite grace gave me a vision. And while the interpretation eluded me, and may still elude me to its full extent, I feel God wanted me at least to write it down.

This is the full account of the "Prayer Vision" and how it was discerned to me, or at least what it has meant to me personally;

Amazing as it is in the case of my life, whenever I feel I have little desire to do something of which I am actually being told to do either by God, a parent or someone in authority over me, a nudging by my own laziness or hard-headedness seems to prompt me first not to do it, certainly to moan and groan about it? And actually, most of the time, these thing's I finally reluctantly do anyway actually after the fact materialize into a realization that they are probably good for me in the first place. Usually, these particular activities in these particular moments, are exactly what I'm supposed to do, and as it turns out, that in many cases it would seem that God has something very good in store for me if I decide to do them anyway!

So was the case of a particular invitation to a men's prayer meeting at 6:30 am on a Tuesday morning when I really had little or no desire to get out of bed. It was my first of such prayer meetings, and I didn't feel particularly at home, or did I expect to get anything too significant out of it. I have never been much of a praying person, having never been taught, (Catholic school upbringing), and if I was, I certainly was either not paying attention, or didn't remember.

But with much prompting, mostly by my mother, I decided to go. Not much to it a group of guys get together to share some breakfast, donuts, and coffee, and talk about things that seem to be of concern or struggle to each of them? As for me, in this particular time of my life, the crisis was on such an upward swing, you would think my crisis engine was spinning at ten thousand rotations per second! So to say the most I didn't seem to get anything from it, but the donuts were good. As it began to draw to an end the men decided, or maybe this is a regular occurrence, to close with a prayer, and in typical fashion, I closed my eyes, and maybe even started to listen agreeing with the prayers of the leader or other men as they, in turn, chimed in.

At this particular moment a different man than the first spoke and for some unknown reason, I turned my head without opening my eyes to look at the man speaking. This was a bit unusual for me because it wasn't like I was expecting to see anything in the darkness of my closed eyes. But to my amazement I did see something; coming from the direction of the man I was looking at, I could see in my closed-eye landscaped darkness a distinct wave action emanating from his direction.

Pulsating waves from a distinct point, his point, and radiating up and out, almost in a wave-like fashion of a pond or something, except still dark, I almost had the impression I was looking into a dark pool on a clear dark night, and someone was throwing stones into the pond. Waves moving out, but mostly up. These waves created an almost uniform undulation in the blackness of my eyesight, or lack thereof, creating only slight shades of black with very dark grays, yet clearly crest with lighter highlights one would see in clear ripples moving across a surface of the water at night.

I sat there and stared for quite a moment, which seemed like a long moment. Thankfully the man leading the prayer was a bit long-winded because I had time to turn my head to the direction of the other men, those next to the one I first noticed, the others to my other side, and even the leader in front of me, realizing that each was creating his own sets of waves. They were each on their own pulsating tempo, and with their own strengths, and as I sat in amazement, I began to realize that all of the wave patterns were slowly starting to assimilate into one, a single greater and very directed large wave, and this wave was pulsating at such an intensity that I could almost physically feel the pulses in my body, especially as I became aware that they were coming. Kind of like the soft reverberations a person feels from the base during a concert.

The wave continued and that was the only thing I could see in the vast darkness of my closed-eyed vision, but suddenly the enormous wave began to lose strength and eventually dissipated to nothing, only moments shortly prior to the conclusion of the prayer. I later shared the sight, vision, whatever, with my then teacher and very close friend Robert, but the meaning of the experience was not clearly brought to me until much later, even days and weeks.

God spoke to me through many words including verbal confirmations, spoken words, written words, preached, taught, every sort of very Godly people and friends in my life, and even the "still soft voice" that I should listen to the most, but which admittedly, I ignore more than hear myself.

In clarifying the vision, God basically said; "All that you see, all that you touch, all that you hear, taste, smell, feel, is not the real world, but the things you don't see, feel, touch, hear, or taste are truly the real things."

And as I pondered this, He spoke to many other examples and how they play into the spiritual battles that are constantly waging around us unseen! "For we do not battle against flesh and bone, but against principalities and forces unseen..."

For example; you are created in the image of God, and with that, fortunately also comes a responsibility of being a creator yourselves. That one fact being "creator" sets you apart from all other creations. The entire universe was set into creation with the spoken word! You confess your salvation before Man with the spoken word. You will be accountable for every "Word" that is uttered out of your mouth, and many more examples of where the word; "Word" is mentioned as a powerful and creative force.

Now scientists will tell us that energy cannot be created or destroyed and if this is the case, what happens to all of those spoken words that we have ever uttered? Do they just disappear, or as scientists may state with energy, and maybe even God verifies (as if He needs to verify anything a man should speculate), that it just keeps going, ever-weakening in effect, weaker and weaker as they dissipate, in essence, settling into the environment around precipitating over time, less of an influence on the things around them then they may initially, yet half of even a very small amount is still half?

Never quite gone, always having some effect on the world around us, our family, friends, this chair, ourselves, forever accountable! So maybe like the prayer, our words are real things, animate, real creations in an unseen world, but because we don't see the effect on the in-animate, on that rock, or on that wall, we assume they have no effect. But the effect, like the real action in the experiential world, is a real effect in the unseen world.

How significant in our real or seen world are the effects of things that are unseen? The effect of love, hate, slander, radiation, poisonous gas, phobia's, too much sun, too little sun, a flirting glance from a beautiful woman, a judgmental look from a boss or teacher, the poker face or lack thereof, a smile, a babies breath, a lover's scent, the statement to a child "your stupid", your pretty, your fat, you're a genius, being told you have cancer, or that someone is proud of you? Many of these types of unseen entities, words, waves, can have a life-changing effect for years even into generations, perhaps much more permanent than even a baseball bat to the same head.

Well, if that be the case, maybe we can take it one step further, and when we do something we know is wrong, is it possible that it's not just an arbitrary event. Often believing that if we don't hurt anyone, or nobody sees the harm in it, that it doesn't have a lasting and permanent effect?

Maybe, just maybe, we are creating entities in the spiritual world, real anomalies that just kind of gather around us, almost like spiritual dark balloons, or bricks, or something maybe even more dark, sinister, and not so desirable, that over time, and with enough accumulations, these things have the ability to isolate us from all who we love; God, our spouses, our children, everything good in the world even ourselves. We become enveloped and saturated with dark!

A single glimpse of porn may not lead to a divorce, but coupled with many visitations to internet porn sites, might later facilitate a justification of dabbling in chat, and even later maybe a secret meeting with some other lonely darkened soul looking for companionship or something, sitting in the same dilemma not knowing where to look or at what. We might just find ourselves completely surrounded and engulfed in these dark bricks or dark balloons to the point where we can hardly breathe, divorce not only becomes a viable option but the only choice!

We can find examples of this in all forms of short-lived gratification; drugs, hate, theft, alcohol drinking, sexual promiscuity, self-mutilation, overeating, all forms and kinds of sin, perpetrated against ourselves, creating around us an atmosphere of darkness and seclusion that may ultimately result in murmuring, blaspheming, pride, even suicide, the ultimate act of self-hatred! When all is dark, why continue? How sad that in most cases it was our own hand that built every dark brick, every dark crude oil-drenched mouthful, every bit of straw and mud, one spoon, one puff, one look, one shackle, one piece of stone at a time.

But praise Jesus when He says; "If you ask for forgiveness, I will place that sin as far away as the East is from the West!" Why does God have to move it away if it doesn't exist, if it is just some insignificant, invisible event in the past? Is He actually picking up something real and moving it?

But if one is true, could the opposite be true also, we should also examine the other side of the coin; Love! When we love our neighbor as ourselves, when we do a kind unselfish thing for our neighbor, our spouse, our children, strangers, our enemies, say a good or kind thing, speak an uplifting word even to ourselves in the mirror, maybe we are creating something substantial in the heavenly realm, something that has a lasting effect on the entire universe, something that can't be taken from us, something that we may even take with us in death?

Acts of obedience, when done for the Heavenly Father all have to be acts of love! Maybe we are building that spiritual temple that mansion that we, as created in the image of God, may possess also.

"For all the commandments, the greatest of these is love."

When we speak of Jesus, we minister or witness is it not said; "this can only be done through the Holy Spirit, which is Love in us." And is it also said that; "Love can only come from God!"

Maybe this is what is meant by; "storing your treasures up in heaven, where there is no rust, no worm to eat, or no thief to steal. For where your treasure there your heart will be also."

What a wonderful thought; to think that with each loving, kind, or good word spoken from our mouths, or the very actions of our lives we are creating something total and indestructible, indestructible in the unseen but real universe.

If the spoken word has such creative power, and love has its own creative manifestations, what about the combination of the two, resulting in praise and worship? What a powerful effect that the combination of these two creative powers manifests, and it is no wonder why the Lord basks in the praises of His people! Did he not say that even the angels stop and take notice, and God himself turns His face towards the praises of His people!

He created us in his image and then so desires for us to express ourselves in a way that demonstrates our true Master's design.

It becomes a bit scary to think that with every action, that might not be particularly of God, we can be creating a negative influence in the universe as well.

This realization manifested itself into a bit of release from me also, into the realization and significance of forgiveness when a person creates a significant amount of black entities around themselves, they begin then to become trapped in their private dark hell they have created, it becomes impossible for them to find love or have a loving act in that secluded place. As if the darkness blocks the light from getting in. Forgiveness is, in essence, a sledgehammer to knock down the wall of darkness we all create around us. I have often heard it said; "You cannot find true love in another unless you first find it in yourself."

It also became understandable how flesh, or the desire for the darkness, would dominate in such a situation, and the spirit desiring good would be weak or nearly non-existent. I often wondered how some self-proclaimed people of faith regardless of the religious name could confess Christ or God, and still act so dark, with hate, theft, or contempt towards each other?

I say a release for me, because when I think about a person engulfed in a quagmire or dark slime, built up with many layers of bricks, mortar, and filth, that has accumulated over years, months, days, or even a moment, it takes away the personal aspect of their attack, and kind of shows me where the real blame for this poor soul rests, making it much easier to hate the sin but love the sinner! To forgive!

Forgiveness an act of love, and the very act of placing away from us, in the same way, God places away from himself sin; it is so comprehensible how the effect of the sin loses its hold on our immediate world. And while we often feel at the time, we are doing someone else such service or a self-sacrificing act, in reality, we are doing something for ourselves that not only benefits us directly but also the world immediately surrounding us.

In this way, we also set down a hedge of protection around

our family and friends and everyone we pray for, forgive and love. We build fortresses around all of the people we love, making it possible for them to experience love much easier than without our efforts. All of this through the miraculous gift of mercy, forgiveness, grace, and love; the greatest gift of God! We in effect spent the shades of all our homes to the light, what chance does dark have in its desire to attack?

So while I was experimenting with prayer as a means to see if it had any effect on people's lives I was working with, on the opposite side of the world, Anna was experiencing the real effect that merely mouthing the words of forgiveness both towards others and to oneself has. Michelle gets completely healed of stage four blood and bone cancer, forgiveness is spoken, the light turns on and sickness flees! I'm saying into darkness as waves in a pond, eating donuts?

Turning on lights have the effect of bathing the entire house with light, a sort of flash of Godliness or goodness occurs, and in essence, darkness has no choice but must flee. A likewise knowledge of where the darkness flees to become evident and deciding as a person, I am not going to go crawling into the shadows just to be bitten by the bugs, seems to be a logical next step?

So is it with sicknesses removing the darkness that you have surrounded yourself with allows then the light to shine through and the sickness must flee.

A Direction is revealed, the direction of the Attack! Essential information if you are even going to contemplate any kind of defense or for that matter a counter-attack. The direction of an attack is basically an evaluated essence of Victory. A target for punches is revealed.

Analyzation of any injury starts and rests upon the shoulders of a proper interpretation of where it comes from.

The great part about this investigation as to how the creature come came in, rests on the fact that it is usually obvious! With the raccoons, it is clearly obvious, with a probable trail of destruction and garbage right to the window sill!

The child coming back from school; the window is the direction of the school, she came home from school. Again obvious! Not so obvious when you are dealing with an injury or something as complex as depression or is it?

When a person is afflicted with anything, regardless if it is a direct physical attack, a systemic realization of something wrong, or a spiritual manifestation of fear or anxiety, the answers to the questions of where it comes from ALWAYS presents themselves. We merely must examine what we were doing at the time of the specific injury or problem, and if this is not clear, what we are thinking, or dreaming, or experiencing, at the very moment of the attack. In every case, the answer to what direction the attack is coming from is made apparent to us. If it isn't clear all we have to do is ask God.

If for some reason the meaning of information seems to elude us, yes we can always ask God. "We have not because we ask not," or so it was said in the Bible by James.

Many spiritual, and even new-age teachers would agree that words have power, and speaking the words with intent will produce results, and in this case of wisdom. I have from time to time asked people who have suffered from this or that affliction to recall what they were doing or further what they were thinking at the time of the attack, but the specifics, especially when linked to severe trauma, or any memory whatsoever was gone. In this particular case asking God for wisdom usually results in a direct and usually clear image or dream appearing in the person's mind. This intuition or miraculous insight, I have found is often exactly tied to the issue at hand.

The good news if these are truly dark spirits that are behind these issues, then one thing is certain, they want to be seen. It grants them no benefit in this or the supernatural world for their dark act to go on unnoticed, as a matter of fact, the more people that know, the greater the fear, the better. This is why they always tip their hand.

Maxine

Mornings light glistens on the edges of the reality, each of its own highlights themselves presenting upon display for yet another of the numerous gifts the God of Life has so graciously given all of us. For I am but here at this moment to observe each of their slender created hues of a masterpiece design, perfect and balanced, they call with whispers of praise; "See me for I exist." Why? But if not for one reason in this moment of time and space, for me alone to see them.

I answered a call to help a woman who hadn't been out of her home in nearly a year. When I showed up at her house, the prescription I had received was written instructing me as I practiced in this particular time physical therapy specifically instructed in peoples homes, usually because they are unable to leave home and must receive their care there. My specific instructions to help this particular person, this patient with her gait strength, stating simply that she needed help with fall risk outside her home.

Before coming I had spoken to her on the phone at which

time she was adamant about needing to know the exact moment I was approaching the door because she stated that she preferred to open the door and allow me to just walk in rather than me knocking or ringing the doorbell. She further explained that this always causes her to become immediately scared and once this happens chances were she would probably not even answer? This was a bit curious, but over the course of thirty years I have seen many such abnormalities, so be it, I did as she asked.

Entering her apartment I was immediately greeted with a sense of home as the soft light and cozy atmosphere she had assembled around her gave the impression of a person who surrounds herself with peace and love, displaying many objects that comfortably speak of a life engulfed with family, children, and goodness. At least that is how it appeared. Upon walking up to the apartment I already had an opportunity to observe the outside sidewalks and terrain around the walkways, seeing nothing unusual that might present itself as an irregular or an immediate danger, so I asked her why she didn't go outside.

Upon entering I observed that while she held on to various pieces of furniture including the walls, she clearly walked with enough stability that a walker was not even a necessity, and that seemed to match the observed placement over in the corner of the room being casually used right now as a coat rack. The majority of the walking she was doing, basically, was holding on mainly for confidence, more so than actually needing to support herself, for the most part, she walked throughout the apartment with good strength, adequate speed, and more than sufficient balance.

This sweet woman we will call Maxine, quickly stated that she hasn't gone out for over six months now, and probably thinking about it, it might even be close to a year.

"You live alone?" I asked.

"My daughter," she says; "Comes and visits me almost every day bringing everything I need, and other than the cat, or going to the doctor on occasion, I never venture outside."

So I asked her why what happened did she fall? But she assured me that she had never fallen inside or outside but got to the point in her existence inside the house where she didn't trust going outside, mainly because she didn't sleep at night and often in the morning she was so tired, her balance was at risk.

I went on to ask her about her sleep and she shared that she had repeated anxiety attacks every night for the last fifteen years, needing at least three sleeping pills to get even a little sleep, this left her often in the morning so tired she could hardly move. This is a common occurrence, sleeping pills while they allow a person to get what feels like sleep, the body does not come into a place of true rest, and she was probably experiencing a sort of exhaustion by the early morning.

At this point it was so long since she had been outside, she was flat out afraid of even the idea of going outside. This fear even manifested so much in Maxine that she was not even willing to answer the door, thus prompting her to speak to me on the phone, needing to know when I was going to walk up, because she would have to unlock the door, telling me to let myself in, as she stood in the corner hoping it was actually me entering. The only other person who came was her daughter and she entered in pretty much the same way.

Maxine had allowed fear to take hold of her world, limiting her to the point where it affected her health. Giving her exercises or instructions to help her get stronger, while it may affect her overall balance, resulted in nothing more than placing a bandage on a bug bite but then letting the bug remain where it is. And since she had no clear deficit, except possible fear, this would only amount to providing her a sort of home personal trainer, something her insurance clearly discouraged.

I suggested if she wished to solve her problem of not being able to go outside she must conquer her fear. She was willing to try but clearly stated her doctor had told her years ago that there was nothing she could do about the anxiety attacks and she just needed to learn to live with it.

Start the program; turn on the light, find out where the attack is coming from and close the window.

We set up a scenario where she imagined an onset of fear, by describing someone coming in the middle of the night and suddenly knocking on the door. This immediately precipitated the same fear reactions she felt at night, but with this exception, we went through a practical and useful solution, in this case, I knocked on the door and she told the person knocking to go away or she was calling the police!

We knocked again on the door, she commanded the person to leave in a clear loud voice, and her own fear again left! I knocked again and told her this time just tell the fear to leave. The fear immediately left again.

After the third or fourth time I said; now I am going to open the door and we are going to go outside; "when you feel fear tell it to leave!" She said she would try. We opened the door she immediately said; "Leave, for God's sake, leave!" looked at me with a smile and stepped out through the door.

She promptly turned to me and asked if she needed her walker? I asked; "Are you afraid you are going to fall?" She shrugged and I said; "Tell the fear to leave!"

She did and smiled and started walking down the walk. We walked up and down the sidewalk for the next twenty minutes and then back to her apartment, in which I hugged her for everything she taught me and said I will see you in two days for your next visit. If you want we will work on your anxiety attacks!

The daughter called the next day asking what did I do for her, what exercises did I give her because her mother had been calling everyone she knew asking them to come over and walk with her outside, not even wanting to take the walker. I told the daughter, to be honest, I gave her no exercises at all.

The next visit I asked her if she still wanted to work on the anxiety attacks, she said maybe but she didn't think it would help, the doctors said there is no cure for anxiety.

"You still pay that doctor," I jokingly said? "Anybody who

tells you there is nothing they can do for you but you still pay them or keep going to, seems to me is like going to a mechanic with a funny sound in your engine, being told he can't fix it, pay him anyway and then keep going back for the same advice?"

She laughed.

So what shall we do about these anxiety attacks?

"Find out where the attack is coming from, pick up a weapon, and fight."

I went on to say; "let's examine what happens the next time you have an anxiety attack because we need to find out what is going on?"

"Perhaps it would be best to leave the room go into another room, and do something that will inject goodness into all of your senses such as read a book, pet the cat, eat a chocolate, whatever, do something good that fills your eyes, ears, and senses with goodness, and I believe you will scare away the anxiety attack."

"But do me a favor, take a small paper and write down exactly what you were thinking about, feeling, or experiencing no matter how insignificant at the very moment you first started to feel the anxiety come on or the moment you wake."

She quickly said; "I don't need to write it down, because I can tell you right now what it is, it is the same thing I was thinking at the moment of every anxiety attack I have experienced for the last fifteen years. It is always the same."

"I worry about my son. His wife is a witch and she hates me so much she refuses to allow me any contact with my grandchildren."

Window found!

"Does your son know you've been waking up every night worrying about him?" I ask again to make sure she sees the window.

"What, and pile my problems on his already huge pile of problems?" she almost angrily snaps back at me.

I redirect so she sees the cause and asked her; "Can you solve any of those problems when you are sitting or lying there?"

She says; "Of course not, I can't help him with any of his

problems, he never listens to me anyway?"

"How does that make you feel, that you can't help him?" I asked again.

"Sad, I wish I could help him."

"It makes you sad or it makes him sad?" I ask.

"It makes me sad, of course, he has no idea I am waking up." She says further; "You keep implying I need to tell him this, burden him with more problems, how his mother is having sleepless nights?"

"No" "I think you need to stop burdening YOU with this." "There is nothing you can do to help him, from bed in the middle of the night."

"I'm not saying you should tell him, I am merely wondering after almost fifteen years why and if you have told him?"

"No, and I'm not going to, he has enough to worry about himself. He is such a pussy when it comes to his wife, he won't do anything about it anyway. She has on multiple occasions told him if he doesn't do exactly what she wants she will take the kids and leave."

Attacking creature and direction of attack identified!

"So you have this worry, this problem, this attack, and there is nothing you can do about it, basically you just take it year after year?" I ask as she looks at me with a tear of realization.

"I guess?" she says with little more sadness than expressed a moment before.
Close the window, clean up the mess.

"This is what I want you to do; forgive your son for being a pussy and not standing up to his wife for what is right. Even if it means you are just mouthing the words, say them anyway, out loud so you can hear them yourself."

"What you can do is forgive him for what he did that cause you to worry!" "And forgive yourself for not being able to help, for not standing up to his wife for what is right with his own kids!"

She said it and did what I told her that moment.

"And now most importantly, forgive yourself for being a bad mother, raising a pussy son, just taking it, or whatever else that relates to you having to suffer from this issue for so long.

Say I forgive me."

She did with a bit of a smile.

"The next time it happens, get up and turn on the light, ask God to forgive you and him, that will close the window if it isn't already closed now."

"Tonight as it gets later pick up a book, something good, read it, maybe a warm glass of milk or Chamomile tea, something soothing instead of sleeping pills. Drink a lot of clean clear water all day to flush your system, remember to bless the water with thanks each time you drink. Trust me it helps, and I will call you in the morning." *More light!*

The next morning I called her and she immediately cried out; "wahoo, I had my first full restful night's sleep without pills and any anxiety attack in fifteen years."

I checked on her a week later, she was still sleeping well, walking outside, and having fun telling others her story about how she was cured of something the doctors told her was incurable.

She thanked me over and over, even though I tried to assure her; "Don't thank me, thank yourself for having the courage to face the attack, thank God."

"Thank God," she said.

I Need A Sign

God gives every person alive who chooses to look into the light, signs to show them that He truly fulfills His promises. Rainbows, they are God's gift to all people as a reminder to them that He always keeps His promises. It is no different in healing when people are faced with drastic and dramatic choices, you would be amazed how many people look to God when all else seems to fail. I would think God would have it that we would look to the light long before the skies become so dark?

It is no different in my own life or the majority of the people I have treated, people, in general, seem to have to hit rock-bottom before they are willing to actually make real changes that result in some good and positive directional change in their lives. I must honestly say over the course of my adult life the majority of the greatest and most positive changes in my own life seem to take place on the coattails of calamity.

It is said; *"All things can be turned to good for those who seek God."* It is no different in health, storms, or dealing with attacks, it merely presents opportunities for growth, which by the way is every given day of our life.

Like the rainbow, the statement; "All things can be turned to good for those who seek God" is a promise.

I myself have seen rainbows of all types in the oddest of places when I have been in a place of asking, either looking to God's for help, and then waiting on Him for answers, guidance, and/or help, or merely looking to God in general in my life whether it be in a quest for what He might want from me, or merely in search of goodness, most of the time I merely need to take a mere moment to look. God gave that gift to men way back when He first gave it to Noah, always has, and continues today, for those who first step out into the light, choose to follow, and look in the right direction, promises are delivered.

Which direction should I look, one might ask? Like every road leads to Rome, any direction you look searching for God, if He truly created everything, then one can assume if you are looking for Him regardless of the direction, and you look close enough you will find Him. Lord Kelvin is commonly known for the quote; "If you study science deep enough and long enough, it will force you to believe in God."

I myself have come to realize the deeper I study anything regardless of the direction or fraction of its real existence, the more convinced I become of one undeniable truth, and that is that God must have created it, governs its path, and demonstrates his very fingerprints on every aspect of its creation. Admitting this fact in my own life resulted in a look to God moment, denying it throughout my life, in essence, was nothing short of a denying of God Himself.

And even Einstein said; "Look deep into nature, and you will understand everything better," but what he didn't explain was which direction or what part of everything he was talking about? But if everything can be explained regardless of which direction one looks, because in essence everything that is, is formed from the same base energy materials then the explanation of everything in its totalitarian, all energies being really the same? Einstein would also have us believe; "energy cannot be created or destroyed, it can only be changed from one form to another," another quote. Believing this one must assume that everything means everything, and thus God who we can also assume created and is in everything states; "I Am the alpha and omega, the beginning and the end" is talking about everything, and then by deduction of both quotes, and assuming everything means everything, no other conclusion can be taken then to assume every promise God has made is absolutely true, and will come true.

How do we know it is the right direction though?

The majority of people do not look to God until the situation or issues of the world literally force them to. All forms of storms, afflictions, attacks, or infirmities can be classified into one simple example; children find themselves either by action or directions at one moment or more face down in the muck. When you are face down in the muck there are two choices every individual must choose; either leave their face in the muck give up and die or lift their head up and live?

Any direction if it is in the direction of God, light, love, peace, must be right since all these are basically the same. Lifting the head up is basically lifting it towards God, you are lifting your head up with the choice for life, life is a gift from God and thus you are choosing God, whether you realize it or not.

This upward motion represents a desire to live on and not just give up. Lift your head, look up to God and you are taking the first step onto the path of healing no matter what affliction you are suffering from.

I have also seen it in patients when they have resided themselves to the fact in their minds that they "Are" patients, they seem to give in to a constant fixation with their own health issue, in an almost constant bowing down posture of their conscious spirit, eyes down, sad, and completely negative about their chances to ever get better. For the most part, a person even though they may present all the abilities to improve, dwell on their losses, take on a spirit of doubt, or negativity about any chance for improvement. A constant staring into the shadows seems to occur, perhaps this is the intention of the attacking spirit?

"Look up, up is always good. Lift your face out of the muck!"

Many people believe and often ask the question; "If God is a loving God why does he create the problem, the sickness, the attack, the problems in my life, The muck, I happen to find myself face down in."

Maybe it is because He is a loving God, and He created this reality for us to enjoy? As in all creation, in order for it to have substance, it also casts a shadow. The shadow is not darkness but is often used by the darkness because darkness is so afraid of the light, darkness lurks in the shadows, darkness, and shadows; these are two distinct and different things.

The objects created are not the shadows, but merely cast the shadow as they block out the light. The shadow is merely the area created space subject to reduced or absent light, without physical form, unable to harm you, but it is here that darkness lingers.

The muck is not the enemy, it is merely being used by the enemy to inflict harm. Look to the light, the darkness flees from the light. Add light to your life and the darkness must flee.

Back to the rainbows and God's promises; God keeps all His promises and will show you all the time and whenever you look in the form of signs, visions, dreams, sounds, recollections, rainbows, rainbow-like appearances of colors on objects, angles in their appearance or directed actions, birds, pets, butterflies, snowflakes, healing, and the list goes on and on into infinity. God basically shows Himself in every creation for those who are looking, everything in nature. I guess Einstein had it right after all?

"Ask and ye shall receive, for you have not because you ask not." Believe that you are loved, and as a loving Father, God would hold back no good thing from His child who asks.

I guess this is where so many people fail, especially when it comes to severe injury or diseases, they are so convinced by the world, by the media, by our educational institutions, by the doctors, that certain things are just incurable or permanent, that they are not willing to even ask, or asking represents some kind of hocus-pocus, false hope for a miracle, or worse yet, a defiance of the authorities in place. The majority of the people who walk through the door, while believing miracles do happen, fear they only happen to others and never to them.

Over the course of the last thirty years, I must say, maybe it was seeing or treating so many injured individuals or perhaps being engulfed in the health care system itself, either way, I must say I have seen or heard reported by many of my colleague's reports directly or witnessed almost every sort of miracle, seemingly more and more frequently as the recent years progressed. I must say I have been perplexed myself why some people seem to be miraculously healed with what is said to be incurable afflictions, yet many suffering from the same, also at times who ask, are met with silence or even worsening issues?

People need healing in many different areas of their life, often unaware or worse ignored by their own hearts, and it is in this area that choices are made whether they chose to believe God or believe what they have been told. It boils down to choice, every soul has free will do they choose to listen to what the world has told them, or do they listen to God?

Health, Wellness, Real healthcare, and possibly the God Gene itself is engulfed and dependent upon the realization of God-given truths. It is the application of these truths, within each of us, allowing for the realization of the promised outcomes granted to each of us by the reality of the entire world God has created for us in this life. This totalitarian experience we know as our soul, encompasses our entire life, and if we believe one part of this reality, it is not much of a stretch to believe all of it?

Jesus the son and the physical manifestation of God's own self and made physical is the greatest of these promises, He demonstrated to all of His children the free gift of healing granted each and every one of us. Everyone who was willing to lift their head, or eyes, hear or come, turn towards God, just call, all who were willing to, but for a moment, believe, and look in the direction of God for resolution of the storms from which these afflictions caused them, received healing.

Doing anything with the intention of doing what God would have you do, especially with healing, no matter the situation, storm, or plan, it has within that moment's reality, in its creative momentous perspective, subtlety the result to form a real event in the spiritual realm which is more significant than any physical movements these actions may facilitate in the physical created universe, that is in the physical universe of which your bodies are aware and reside. For the created universe is merely a fraction of the whole in comparison to the physical boundaries of the entirety of creation, our own scientists have stated and presented this repeatedly.

I know this fact myself and always have found it perplexing the thought of so much space and so little actual energy-laden matter. How infinitely small atoms actually are, or viruses for that matter. The vastness of space between planets or stars, or the spaces that science would tell us resides even between the relatively small actual physical boundaries of the components of atoms is almost unbelievable.

An atom is but a conglomerate of energy that comprises the basic unit of fixed material, but science will tell us also that the protons, neutron, electrons are themselves made up of moving components of energy, not solid but more like whirling masses of moving energy plasmas or strings, depending on who you ask, that has been set into motion, not unlike sound. The most basic of these units although find themselves in a formation of a system of energies revolving around each other, complex designs of infinitely small but incredibly strong bonds of cooperating energies that once set into motion are nearly impossible to disturb.

Is the basic point of awareness in the universe and atom, for it had to be set into motion in order for it to be aware of the surrounding space and time? Adam the first man or Atom the first speck of reality both sound like infinite complexities, one mere man in an infinite universe, to start the whole basic human awareness ball rolling. As much as these two words seem to sound slightly alike could we make a correlation between them, especially in the venue of health and wellness, perhaps?

Science will tell us that we are merely a conglomerate of energy; particles of negative charges revolving around positive ones with a few neutral ones thrown in there for good nature. Isn't God wonderful, everything in His creation from the largest to the smallest mimics each other, and ultimately Him, as to place His perfect design or His fingerprints on everything we may take the time to look at, and then hopefully give Him the glory, or at least recognition for this creation?

In my own observations positive particles or in this cases people with truly positive spirits, those who have a Good God dwelling spirit within, rest in a balance of secure stability knowing where they are, and more importantly where they are going, having a sense of balance in the cosmos. Neutral particles can come in close proximity to the positive ones, close but not quite touching, there is no fear, no repulsion, just calm acceptance with a mutual dance of a subtle rotation. Their relationships, even though seemingly held together with threads of a seemingly insignificant and immeasurable force, this force although seems to be blessed with energies of unfathomable consequence, as though the creator himself placed an enormous amount of importance that these bonds, the same force when split would produce enough power to topple all the creations of men.

But not so with the negative ones that circle at a distance, always in motion, unsure of where they are at any particular time, flying around in multiple looping chaotic ovals that speak more of irregularity and nervousness than anything remotely stable. These small almost inconsequential particles and I say almost, because each while taken on its own merit from a worldly standpoint, seem unimportant, being tiny, easily replaced, and prone to chaotic and irrational behavior. They are constantly jumping around from one place to another in a haphazard exchange of static irritation. The energy exchange of this static manner is minor on a one-to-one basis, requiring these little pathetic particles to join forces with many of their cohorts in order to issue any kind of measurable effect. The contrary is their positive brothers, when they split or separate from their created partners enormous energies are released. The negative ones must join in an incalculable quantity of others to make an effect that might mimic the power of the positive ones, such as seen in a lightning bolt, even a small discharge from the nucleus of the positive ones has a broader and more permanent effect on its surroundings when splits occur.

And what is further interesting is that the negative particles are not repelled by the positive ones, no the negative ones flee from the positive ones, because the positive particles remain stationary and it is the negative particles that leave. *"And darkness looked upon light comprehending it not, darkness fled!"*

Let us suppose that these particles are nothing more than the composites of electromagnetic oscillations, as science would have us believe so, which is the very same kind of energy that makes up the sound. And to further stretch our limit of faith in their suppositions, science would have us believe that these incredibly small particles which relative to their size orbit at incredible distances from each other; It has been supposedly scientifically proven, for example, if a standard proton of a nucleus of an atom was merely the size of a basketball and it sat in Chicago, the closest electron would be the size of a pea and be the distance to Kansas City away, but this figure too, has changed from year to year? But what is a strange fact is that somehow they are being held together by some immeasurable force, attractions so strong that they can form bonds that are strong as diamonds, making them somehow also impenetrable to a blending of other unwanted visitors of the same energy makeup, even though these large gaps, these pea-sized so-called insignificant creations.

The very bonds of the positive ones, the likes of which when mere grams are split, not destroyed, but their initial bond split, forms altered, will discharge energy of a caliber so magnificent it can take out entire cities of things man built. It is material the size of a penny that can fuel atomic bombs. *"What God has brought together, let no man bring apart!"*

And all of this magnificent power is a result of something equivalent to the spoken Word. Wow, if the Bible is merely the writings of men, what genius that these men, with their limited scientific accumulated knowledge, for they knew all of this without the aid of modern instrumentation and centuries of learned reference that the universe was "Spoken" into creation. So Moses without the advantage of thousands of years of our so-called evolved intelligence was able to guess that everything was created from the sound when he wrote; "God said let there be...", and we are supposed to believe this was a random guess on his part and not inspired by God Himself, I think not!

Everything that is seen, touched, smelled, tasted, or felt can speak to the glory of God if one will just take the time and look close, even science, even health.

Infirmities of all types, whether they be sicknesses, injuries, or afflictions, whether they are the attacks of a moment, repeated momentary attacks, or even those that can last a lifetime, all are attacks from the outside. The awareness of these, a clear eye needs to be placed back on them to understand them, learn from these experiences, and overcome, this is the path to wisdom. To do this you will need to relearn what has been taught and more importantly what is believed about these storms.

Over the course of the next few months, I began to see a distinct change in the way the patients reacted and healed. People would commonly comment about various aspects of the healing process they until recently either didn't witness or just didn't experience because it wasn't there.

God teaches those who ask about storms in the form of experiences, visions, or dreams, and as in my own case not long after that, the Word comes in.

Let us examine for a moment the true nature of storms.

While storms are the attacks perpetrated upon large groups of individuals and areas of God's creations, sicknesses, and afflictions are the storms that are perpetrated against the individuals singularly and specific for each of us, granting our own momentous opportunities to overcome and continue down the path of the journey He intended in the life He gave each of us.

They are like hurdles in a race, each provides an opportunity to jump over and continue down the path before you. Some afflictions, like some storms, even like some battles in wars, are physically not able for an individual to overcome, and it is for these individuals and but for God, the One and Only, resulting decision making Entity, the ultimate decision making finality, the Alpha and Omega, of creative placement in the garden perspective, a realization of when a spirits time within their given soul needs to leave the human awareness physical so-called reality realm and return to the real and totalitarian primarily spiritual, completely enlightened realm of the heavenly existence, those either with God or away from Him, depending upon your own choice as a spirit.

God would have that every one of us would get out of the boat and come to Him, for it is in this moment that we do not calm the storm, it is in this moment of water walking that we do not need to. The storm itself cannot kill us, only when we do nothing like sinking into the abyss as a desperate loss of all hope, a dismal solution can.

We all would love to see a sign, but for those who are willing to believe that one is out there, we are immediately and completely bombarded with signs that every real thing is a sign.

Sicknesses Are Simple Things

Diseases; Such Small Things

Life can be such an experiential place of observation granting us experience even if only in our dreams today, granting confidence for the challenges and obstacles we may face tomorrow, so was it for a young pre-med student early in his education when it came to germs and diseases.

Enter Dr. J; like many other pre-med students often an opportunity is given for small part-time assistant positions where some low-paid assistance is given to one or more doctors doing research on campus, as a way to earn a little of the education costs. Dr. J was a researcher of amoeba's, but not just any old amoeba, but a particular one that when activated was fatal to humans, as he put it; "finding itself in the food or stomach and then boring its way up into the brain of the person, multiplying, and the result was death, no cure." "You needn't worry," the doctor quickly added, "these amoebae are all around us, in the lakes we swim in, in and on the fruit we eat, and the majority of the time they just exist and never harm us." "But once in a great while, once in about a hundred million, or maybe a hundred trillion if you are counting them, one of these little creatures will just decide to go crazy and attack, no rhyme or reason behind it, it just attacks and that's it."

Dr. J's job was to try to figure out why these would suddenly attack? He assured me they were not contagious, nor did I need to worry about handling the many test tubes and instruments he had cleaning on a daily basis.

I didn't realize until years later the significance of such statements.

A year later I found myself volunteering in a Medicine Testing laboratory in Leeuwarden, Holland where I tested medicines and combinations of medicines against various strains of extremely dangerous and infectious diseases, among others, live samples of "The Black Death." The lead Dr. H a very renowned and confident instructor assured me that as long as I was careful and followed her instructions when it came to disinfecting the instruments with a flame I was completely safe from catching any of the sicknesses. No gloves, no mask, no hazmat clothing was worn by her, myself, or anyone else. Nobody ever got sick.

Dr. H taught me something very important and profound;

"That germs are so small and weak they can hardly move around through space, and mostly have to be attached to fluids, in a very self-supporting and transportation dependent way. And viruses even more so are so fragile that they cannot even live outside the extremely stable and temperature constant environment we provide in our cells. She said when handling these creatures, whether testing, treating, or eliminating, the only thing you have to fear is fear itself.

Sicknesses of all kinds manifest themselves in the form of attacks, whereby most people know the very moment usually the very first feel they may have experienced the attack.

So for the case of our study let us assume that sickness and affirmatives are an attack of an outside entity, a spiritual entity, or at least in the majority of their influence they are mostly spiritual and only the slightest bit physical. Then correspondently understanding this is the first step in defeating it, because at the very least it results in turning the light on to the situation, at the earliest point of the attack, when the least effect has already been done.

To understand the nature of healing one must first examine and understand the aspects of exactly what is going on. A person cannot understand, let alone hope to fight a battle if they are looking in the wrong direction or blind to exactly what forces are attacking.

Infirmities of all types, whether they be sicknesses, injuries, or afflictions that can last a lifetime, yet are attacks from the outside. People believed this once and today there needs to be a relearning of what is believed about such things.

We have discussed three examples to describe the nature of sicknesses; the Bully, the Raccoon, and the Spy, a fourth which I will call a mere Hole in the road, amounts to merely that something small and laying in your path, something you can fall into, an event out of your own cause, something placed on your direction you are walking, and usually unseen results in injury, pain, and ultimately destruction of either part of your body or the whole physical self.

The Vision of the Hole in the road;

If one could see disease as it might present itself, one might look at the affliction as if it is a small hole in the road. It is then you the traveler coming along this path, in this new day and a single moment of time, unaware of the hole lurking within a few steps on the path, the one you have chosen or placed upon, inadvertently gets ready to fall in?

Some travelers are brought down this particular path by their own choices, some are led by their parents, some are guided as an opportunity to get to a greater place, some are exactly where they were supposed to be, some are guided by desires that are bad for them and often others around them, but regardless of the circumstances of the particular path choice, the fact of the matter is the hole awaits.

Now, why does the hole exist? The hole may have been created by the careless actions of those before you, it may have been a natural occurrence in the balance of life around you, it may have been a product of your own hands years before unknowing digging, and it may be a trap?

Now in this case what is exactly is the hole, when inadvertently stepped into, possibly causing injury; is the hole the injury, or is it merely the mechanisms used to inflict injury?

When many different persons step along the same path and come to the same hole many individuals fall to the same fate, they step in without noticing it, stumble and even perhaps break their ankle or leg from the fall, their body starts working at less than optimal level, a feeling they often associate with becoming ill, but often this change is merely the bodies own attempts to rectify the local damage as soon as possible without allowing further damage to occur.

Some overcome the fall by catching themselves with the strength and skill usually granted them by training or youth, some are even given the natural gifts to overcome physically such challenges immediately, some fall but their bodies are strong enough or flexible enough to absorb the blow.

Some are carefully watching enough their steps to avoid the small places where the dangers lie, and some can jump over when the obstacle appears.

So is the hole the injury? If so why did the hole not hurt the one who jumped over?

No, the hole is not the sickness, it was merely being used by the spirit of injury as a mechanism to inflict its task, like a wolf waiting in the hole for an unsuspecting traveler to venture by. An angry but little wolf, hiding in the recesses of holes that have been deposited in the path of God's unknowing little path walkers.

Of course, the smaller, the less experienced, or the more feeble the people, the elderly, or people who have fallen many times before, the more susceptible they are to injuries, the easier prey for the wolf.

The little wolf is injury and is a coward, he hides in the recesses of the dark place, waiting and hoping to sink his hungry teeth into the Godly gift of the leg, or more vulnerable body part that may present itself.

One may ask why does God allow the hole to exist, but I think we all know this answer, holes in the road are a product of us not taking care of the gifts God has already given us, misuse, or even sabotage by others intent of setting traps or hoping for another to fall.

No, the hole is not the problem, the little creature, the little nuisance, a little bug for some, with aspirations of being a fierce wolf to others, he is the problem. The hole merely is the potential for a problem, a potential is not a problem, it is merely what might occur if one falls in? But if a person doesn't fall regardless of the size of the said hole then no accident has occurred, thus "nothing" happens. So by deductive reasoning, if the potential for injury is the sickness, the storm, the disease, and a person has a fall, comes down with it, catches it, or takes it upon themselves, before it can become realized before it is realized it is unrealized!

The Hole is not Everything, as a matter of fact, if he is not everything, and everything comes from God, then the hole is what is left, and that means the fall is nothing. Take away everything and all you have is nothing. But can nothing hurt you? When nothing represents a hole in the road, or better yet a fall into a hole, it can definitely hurt you! That is if you fall?

If God has been true to his Word, and He always is, then we should merely have to look to our surroundings for the solution to our issue, be it the hole or the pesky little wolf bite. Step over, climb over, go around, or take a leap of faith.

The hole should be easy, use everything given to us in the immediate proximity to overcome the obstacle at hand whether it be among our own God-given gifts; strong legs, quick healthy reflexes, sharp reasoning, or sharp clear eyes, good healthy voice, or even material that is within our accessibility to overcome the obstacle.

Living in the Southwest on the edge of town one has come into contact from time to time with Javelinas in the yard eating the plants. And while for the most, they are docile and harmless, except to the plants, they can from time to time decide to attack, especially dogs or other animals they may feel are threats. But anyone who has lived in this area long enough would tell you, that all you need to do to get them to leave and leave quickly is go out and make a little noise, the louder the better. A good loud spoon hitting a pan is usually sufficient to get them all to run for the hills.

Most of the time a good strong voice is all we need to scare away such a pest. As simple as it seems just telling it to leave especially in the name of God, is usually enough.

I always wondered why people for centuries would say; "Gezondheid" which is basically "Blessed Health" in Dutch, "Na Zdrowie" in Polish mean "To Health," or often also "Bless you" or "God Bless You" when someone sneezes? Is it perhaps because people have known for centuries that the sneeze may be a warning or an impending or instantaneous small attack against an individual, and your body is warning you of it as it attempts to discharge it? So the person wishing health, as a matter of fact, God blessed health, when the sneeze occurs, actually sends health to the sneezing individual and into themselves. It has been scientifically proven that praying or wishing health to others, improves your own health immediately.

The resulting wish; a person is bathed with the sound of another person's blessing. These good sounds go in and on every aspect of the person who is sneezing, and darkness flees!

But I have seen that the majority of the people when it comes to healthcare just climb down and try to crawl through the hole, doesn't seem like the most sensible course of action, but how many of us sometimes foolish acting kids seem to choose the most dangerous and impracticable course of action over and over again, instead of just walking around. Then we wonder why we just keep getting a bit over and over again?

Only Chose Good?

Ok, so the fall into the hole represents the injury, what then? What do you do after the fall, the event, the poor traveler steps into the hole and gets bit?

Turn on the light, chase away the wolf, and clean up the mess of the storm. The cleaning is the treatment after the affliction. While we will touch on treatment in this book, treating yourself as God would have you treat will be examined in the next one; Treat Yourself "For God's Sake".

As you may have noticed Jesus always followed up every healing with some kind of action; *"pick up hour mat and walk, go wash in the Jordan, report to the teachers of the temple, go..."*

This is real therapy.

You must not only fight, resist, but also treat in the same perspectives and directions that you were created, injured, or attacked, if you want good or godly results, you must use good and godly instruments.

If you want good and Godly results you must move in a good and Godly direction. Upward works, moving towards the light, these can never be bad, and definitely asking for help from Him who is qualified and wanting to help. When people tell you that you must stop any good or natural applications or they may contradict the direction of the treatment you are receiving, then I would wonder about the intended direction these doctors or agents are advising? If they don't want you to go in the direction of good, light, pure, clean, then what direction are they advising you to go?

If you want good and godly results you speak and hear only good and godly words, sounds, perspectives, and plans.

And if you want a good and godly result you must bath your eyes with light and images that feed your soul with the warmth and love of this good and godly creation.

That seems like a lot of things a person must do and extremely limiting regarding the world as a whole when it comes to trying to limit what direction you go or what instruments you might use along the way, but even the very sights and sound, even your very words along the way, provide an almost limitless abundance of good and Godly material when it is with faith being used.

It always boils down to one simple fact; free will. You always have the simple choice to choose in every aspect around you, in this case, whether or not you wish to heal?

Basically these are all the same but for the purpose of explanation and future reference we will use all of them when describing the nature of each of these attacks, and then relate them to sicknesses or injuries in order to later reference them for further understanding of how to recognize them, and what to do, when the attacking afflictions have been defeated?

Warriors, Come Out And Play

"And Jesus asked him saying, what is thy name? And he said Legion; because many devils were entered into him." Mark 5:9

Accident or example, why this particular possessed man did Jesus ask? It is clearly documented that Jesus cast out demons in many people. Even the Pharisees admitted it with their own accusations when they accused Him of casting out demons in the name of demons, as in Matthew 12:24.

But why was this particular man commented on, noted, and described, not only in one but two Gospels? Was it perhaps to teach? God doesn't just teach with a single action, but with His entire creation, enveloped in every documented event, there is teaching within teaching, within teaching, within an entire philosophy. Is that not so God? Where can we not look in His entire creation, and ever finding more examples of His beautiful creation, evidence of teaching, as we peel back the layers, like a majestic onion?

No, the demon just didn't give a single name or even many, Jesus knew this, He wanted the demon to reveal important information about the structure and even the makeup of our enemy. He solicited out all the information He wanted to be known, like interrogating a filthy spy, He got everything with a single question.

The demon responded "Legion." Not braggingly, almost as if he had the information was ripped from its mouth. "How silly," our Lord must have thought when He considered these creatures that tormented His children. How foolish their plans must appear to Him. What did they think, send an entire legion into this poor soul and perhaps make Jesus seem foolish trying in vain to Exorcise them?

Of course, He knew their names, He recognized their foul stench coming down the path a mile away. He created them, He knew them very well, but we didn't!

In that one statement, the devil's man gave more information away out of its own mouth, then they might have been needed to be revealed by Jesus Himself? Why would Jesus even have to dirty His own mouth by explaining the structure and attack mode of the enemy, when He could have one of the devil's own spill the beans for Him?

Oh, it must have been one angry devil that night, and probably a reckoning paid when the devil found out how one of his underlings spilled the beans with its' big mouth.

Anybody remotely interested in learning about the structure or makeup of the enemy merely has to examine the word Legion, and the picture that word paints; organization, rank, a particular form of attack, strategies associated with it, weapons used, the training and intelligence the participants held, along with the strengths and weaknesses presented with such a military-type organization, all find their way to the canvas layer by layer, brushstroke by masterful brushstroke?

Let us examine for a moment just the structure of sicknesses and their ranks?

The Roman Army was a highly organized very structured ranking of a soldier all methodically grouped for the purpose of following the instructions and eventual wishes of the supreme commander, usually the emperor. This information and if we want to imply intelligence was systematically reduced as it went down the ranks in order to make the most basic orders, the ones at the front lines merely a simple attack, go here or there, stay put. A ruthless horde at the tips of a great spearhead that was the Roman army, that was bent on one goal, to bring under servitude all people who stood before their supreme leader. Capture as much of the free world as they could lay their eyes upon, steal everything of worth to send back as a tribute to the home city and basically to the emperor himself, and finally enslave all who they conquer, killing what those they didn't want, using the rest as slaves to bow down and serve from that time forward, even upon multiple generations.

The smallest group of soldiers eight or so, consisting of the least trained, lowest-ranked individuals was called a "Contubernium" and could be perhaps compared to a small platoon. These front-line troops were often made up of the recently captured of other lands distant, the point being often they didn't even speak the same language but were thrust into a fight for their lives, it was to fight or die often for these basic troops.

Ten of these small groups would be banded together, this larger collection was called a "Century," because it held approximately 100 men, when you counted the support troops and standard-bearer. These men fell under the leadership of one officer a "Centurion," or a captain. Now this one would often be at least be a Roman, having at least some skills in communication, but strategy or any complex thinking was still well above his pay grade with the exception of being a very seasoned and accomplished fighter. One thing he was good at was leading his troops, for discipline was absolute and the orders given by him are followed without question.

Six Centuries together formed a "Cohort," then ten cohorts would be combined to form a "Legion," the basic military unit! This great group of approximately 6,000 men, and was all under the command of few Tribunes, high ranking officials, perhaps like majors, one or two Prefects, or a single Legatus, all under a General, the Proconsul and eventually up to the Emperor.

The army was typically deployed in a three-tear linear system of structure attacks. The first group, "The first in," were called the "Miles," these were fatigue workers, they had other names but the most significant was "Gregorius," which translated; Herd Animals. Represented as I already said by the least trained, most disposable, and least effective individuals.

The second tear was composed of greater skilled, better-trained soldiers, these soldiers, received greater equipment, support, the backing of the army itself, some basic power.

The third group was reserved for the veterans, those with the greatest experience, fighting skill, strength, ability to problem solve, these men were highly favored by the commanding officers, they were the ones that received any spoils of the battle if a spoil was received, but with great reward came great responsibility. If a battle was lost often the blame was placed on these, they were the example made, it was their fault. Of course, the leadership would never take responsibility!

We can learn an enormous amount of information by studying the enemy. The supernatural is always represented in the natural. If we are going to battle the enemy, we should strive to understand him, and one way to do this is to understand the structure of their deployment, their individual pieces, and the possible strengths of attacks whether they be initial or repeated.

First of all the enemy's ranks are divided into organized groups, of which the smallest is deployed into small groups of likewise uneducated, untrained, and ill-equipped entities. These, which are considered almost live-stock-like, don't think for themselves, only react, they are stupid and prone to making dumb mistakes, they have explosive tempers and at any sign or feeling of fear, will go running. They are usually sent in at the very start of a plan to attack to wreak havoc on the would-be victim, sent in without a set idea, no negotiation, just attack regardless of what they come across, a sort of blind hit them anywhere you come in contact sort of intent.

As with the Roman army, and even as seen in the natural, the creatures that have the least abilities, also possess the least intelligence, have the least adaptive skills, and must join forces with large numbers to have any effect on greater skilled opponents. They attack in groups, so unless their numbers are great, they will only pester and never fully attack. Herd animals!

I would equate these with demonic irritations, the kinds that attach themselves on a host or in a particular area, and pester, tempt, oppress, or sicken. These are the kinds that inflict chronic pain or irritation to individuals, maybe even addictions, these are the stupid little ones that do nothing but follow you around and nibble on your ankle all day long. These are the ankle biters!

Spot these cowards, and they are likely to take off merely because of being spotted. Just speaking out loud that you are aware of their mischievous dark nature, maybe enough for them to go running for the hills. It probably wouldn't hurt to send a command after them, as they are running; "Don't come back, I'll line all of you and your buddies and give you a real Godly beating!"

In this example germs would be the inadvertent creatures being used by the sicknesses, the sickness is a spirit driving the germs to attack, the spirit uses the many small creatures, physical objects, or even people to do their destructive tasks for them, in effect they afflict their hosts to then wreak havoc on the target of their attack. Is this perhaps why an amoeba on an Orange would suddenly attack?

Understanding the enemy is the first great step in a plan to defeat it. Sicknesses are the simplest among the spiritual creation. As in the world with various levels of living creatures from the horse to the simple bacteria, why would we think that God didn't create the same diversity so that in the spirit are various levels of functioning spirits from the greatest angels to the simplest small and weakest little basic spirits?

When a third of the angels were deceived and fell this group consisted of all variations of spiritual beings, all now choosing dark, not unlike a random selection of one-third of all living creatures on and in the earth.

As all living creatures of the world were created and placed under the servitude of man, all spiritual creatures were placed under the servitude of the Father.

Many fell! But their numbers are not infinite, they only have so many troops.

People seem to have been programmed or at the very least deceived into believing that sickness and even life-threatening occurrences are somehow like random lurking creatures, some kind of dark beast just outside the limit of their perception waiting to pounce on the unexpected innocents when their guard is down, out of their control, and undetectable yet all-powerful, something to be absolutely eared, at least that is what they would like you to think. Words like diseases or syndrome lurking just outside our awareness to sense, waiting to pounce on unsuspecting and innocent bodies, unable to defend themselves let alone cope with the onslaught.

The Roman army used such tactic of fear, sending word of their onslaught far ahead of their campaigns to the distant lands with their traders and merchants, so when the army even the smallest of bands showed up, they would be so feared that the masses of people would just bow down in submission without even drawing a sword. It was this way that the Romans with so few governing and sustaining troops could put under submission such a vast overwhelming horde of conquered foreign citizens. Fear is everything to them.

Another tactic the Romans would use was that the conquered were somehow inferior in creation to themselves and thus coming into this place of slavery was merely a factor of destiny, because of inferior design?

We too are fed the same dark fake media nonsense that; in some cases flaws like genetically predetermined time bombs sit within each of us that like these ticking time bombs are just waiting to have their own undetectable fuses lit, resulting in the unstoppable and irreversible explosion that destroys bodies, lessen life, and create an environment in which the very soul of our existence seems to be feared or even regretted.

The truth of the matter is actually closer to the model taught than one might imagine; "Infirmity is the lie and but a hue of stain splotched like dirt on the thread of these sicknesses found woven in the tapestry of your destiny that is in question."

Sickness and all forms of Infirmity for that matter are merely small insignificant creatures lurking just outside the limits of our perception, but this is not because it is an inconceivably small creature such as a virus or bacteria lurking ready to attack without mercy, or destined by its shear strength of numbers to eventually overcome, it is merely the event of direct impact followed by the individual decision of being, that this attack has been successful in its attempt to distract us from what God truly had in store for each of us, and that is a purpose and life filled experience in this physical portion of our soul.

Sicknesses and Infirmities are never your destiny but merely unresolved storms you chose to endure rather than overcome. Sicknesses and infirmities are the results of spiritual influences on the simplest of creation, and then our accepted reaction upon ourselves. Therein above rests one of the first lies; if God created each and every one of us perfect then how could He then create us with flaws?

I have witnessed many times in the course of years of treating hundreds if not thousands of individuals, the occasional situation where the available resources granted us within our own bodies seems to rapidly and dramatically reduce to the point where mere daily life almost becomes a difficult and nearly hopeless endeavor. Nowhere is this scene in what appears as a tragedy as when it appears in the life and final days of a chronically and terminally ill child, this leads many who stand just outside the direct influence of this traffic picture wondering about the purpose, if not the

Godliness of such an experience.

Many people are born with flaws not everyone is born perfect, children all the time are born with deformities, issues, syndromes, or even severe sicknesses that lead to very untimely deaths and short lives, I have treated many of these. I have witnessed people who have such poverty or on the receiving end of abuse that the thought of some fair shake in this life seems like a joke to them. This would be a difficult sell to tell such people they have been created perfectly?

Being born with greater challenges either physically or mentally has nothing to do with flaws, every living person has a purpose, a journey to fulfill in the exact place or time God has placed them to experience it. It is, for this reason, I believe, that God has given them everything they need to overcome. Every day is but a new day, and every day another life day for each of us, whether they be eight-plus years or but a couple? If we are to believe any of it then we must also believe the part about being created eternally, and if that be the case when we have lived untold millennia, the thought of this time frame we call our life whether it be many generations in years or but a few days will all seem the same, because to God who is infinite it all is.

Sicknesses, Injuries, Afflictions, or Infirmity's, are all storms, they blow in from afar, cause problems and fear, and in some cases damage even unto death, but for those who overcome the gift of each day is growth.

More and more I began to understand that afflictions seemed to come in waves, attacks, or even in the form of storms, patients would almost without exception have the ability to pinpoint the actual moment they first became aware of an issue, whether it be a direct injury as in some kind of force injury such as a break or accident, or even when more slow-progressing issues occurred, they could even with almost psychic clarity realize the very moment they first became aware that something was amiss?

All infirmities whether sicknesses or injury all result from the same thing, they are the manifestation of storms that occur in people's lives. Like storms, a person must venture into them, whether by their own doing or carried on the back of others that ferry a soul through.

So if we assume sicknesses are like storms then one can assume by looking to the natural as an example to dealing with the supernatural, are we saying many of the storms could be avoided?

Of course. You chose the course especially after you are of the age of accountability, a young teenager or so. But once the storm is being physically experienced by you it is up to you how you are going to deal with it, and this has a profound effect on how much if any damage occurs because of the storm?

There are many examples throughout history where people seem to fall prey to sicknesses and the effects of the storms they feel with throughout the life they have set their own feet into, but yet others seem to go through the same storms unaffected, people are immune or just thought to be strong enough not to so-called catch the sickness others are seemingly powerless to avoid, why is this?

I was often perplexed with the documented fact that people like Saint Francis of Assisi worked with and treated leapers yet never contracted the disease even though at the time there was no effective treatment or medicine for this severe affliction.

Storms do occur, there is nothing you can do except how you choose to deal with them?

Sometimes storms come upon you like a little child running into a bully. We have been brainwashed, taught, and instructed at almost every level from childhood to just take it. Bend over like a slave, give in to the conqueror because ether is nothing we can do, stop trying to even fight yourself, claim it upon yourself and give up, freely give up what God has given each of us; free will?

No more, we say no to slavery, we say no to the attacking bug, we say no to the storm; *"In the name of God, Be still!"*

Peter Colla

Only Prayer and Fasting

It soon became clear that while some sicknesses could be commanded to leave, especially when detected at their very earliest moments, others seemed to take much more effort time or attempts to get them actually to leave and stop bothering the person afflicted.

Almost immediately in the gospels, Jesus gives his followers the ability to go out and do what he has shown them, healing and helping others with their afflictions, then suddenly a man comes to Him or is brought whose son suffers from what appears to be seizures, or perhaps episodes of uncontrollable fits whereby he falls to the ground shaking, apparently convulsing, even hurting himself falling into the fire or water at times?

First Jesus seems to be perplexed by the fact that his followers couldn't take care of this issue and even scolds them to a degree, but then turns to the man and asks him what does he want? I find it a bit rhetorical, but I also realize that this question and many He asks are more for the instruction of myself, the man with the son, His disciples, and everyone else who happens to ever hear about this event in the future, presenting Himself as more a teacher than merely someone delivering treatment and in this case, deliverance to not only the son but the man who obviously must live with this horrible situation? The man obviously loves his son, many would have abandoned such inflicted people, but this man stayed with him, even sought out any help he could find, even when earlier attempts didn't seem to help. Not unlike many who I have treated in the past myself or most who happen to be reading this book?

Jesus then commands the spirit to identify itself, something we will get into in more detail later, but this in itself again is odd, for again as a Master Instructor, He obviously knows the answer to the question before He asks, but wants the information to be told for the purpose of the audience to hear and possibly learn from. We find out it is not only a single spirit but an entire legion? Regardless, Jesus casts it away and then goes on to explain to His followers that; "some such as these can only be removed by prayer and fasting."

The prayer part we got, it is the fasting part that we should examine at this point?

In my limited, fairly regimented, not so faithful in God, and seemingly at the time to be much more constricted when it came to having fun, upbringing, I can say that in and outs of fasting were spoken of little if any, and the actual reasons why someone would fast, how they are to do it, or what exactly the fast was supposed to accomplish was not only rarely explained, for even hardly ever was brought up let alone in the church environment, at least from my experience, to anything at all about the subject. As I delved into the exploration of faith and its possible correlation to healthcare as we know it, I also found very little enlightenment regarding fasting other than a loose association with dieting? For the most part, people just saw it as a process of starving themselves of one or more thing in their life, food being the most common choice, as a way to show obedience to God, or even possibly motivate God in our prayers, as if God could be bought? Seemed to me to be a foolish notion, the God who created everything, would want us to deny from ourselves something we either need or want as a means to express to Him we actually what one Him, want to obey Him, possible prove to Him something He would already know one way or the other, He does know everything?

Back to fasting; but all the teaching or references to at least eating habits seem to point to not overindulging in anything as it was this practice that would put things at least when it came to our own small universes, before God. Information started pouring in about the benefits, almost Godly and miraculous powers that were associated with using, all-natural, whole and complete food, pure waters, herbs, limiting some meats, some people needing some things more than others, all taken in moderate yet almost spiritual considerable fashion?

The spiritual consideration seemed to be the factor that was necessary for the food or product being consumed to have in essence a truly Godly effect. Recently, there has been a number of tests where groups of people all suffering from the same issues placed into blind studies, these are studies where the participants are not told the specifics of the tests being performed on them. These studies would involve one half go them receiving standard treatment, whether it be a drug or procedure, even as aggressive as reconstructive surgery, and the other merely receiving a placebo, yet both would be reported to them that the procedure or effects were superior to what they expected and full success was seen. In both cases, all the subjects would report increases of status even what felt like a miraculous recovery? What was astonishing was when people would be convinced they actually received an operation, and told that it was an enormous success even to the point of a miracle, their bodies would repair themselves and mimic what the person actually believed in their hearts or spirits.

For decades myself, maybe centuries for that matter people have been blessing their food, or at least many do, and it has become so regimented and ritualized that we as people dent really seem to see the significance of this action any longer other than just doing out because we have always done it as our parents had done before us, and theirs before them on and on.

But does the blessing of the food actually do something? Jesus seemed to bless the food and then give it to His disciples, and why would He first bless it if it was for nothing? Nothing only exists in the belief of its negative existence, and God doesn't do anything for nothing, that would basically be the same as producing Light for Darkness? Wait a minute, maybe that's why darkness wants our children or gifts, our very souls because God created them and this beautiful world for that matter for us, and the enemy wants it because he doesn't have anything real for itself, so it wants ours! Our very health!

We have already looked at the positive effects, at least a little, with regards to water, but what about in the foods? We know that water changes on the molecular level for the positive when blessed, and we even know that it changes in such a way that it can actually change the crystallization form, taste, and possibly effect it has on earth, then food also having a large percentage of its mass consisting of water one could assume the same changes would or could occur when it is being blessed as well? But how does this play into fasting?

Recently a program has arisen in which a person could participate in what is called "intermittent fasting," this is an eating program whereby the individual doesn't eat anything for 16 or so hours in the day and holds their meals to within an eight-hour time frame? The fact it is called fasting seems almost supernaturally Godly by my observations, seeing the enormous amount of benefits that a person seems to receive by doing it.

First and foremost, there seems to be a daily resetting of the person's autoimmune system in their body, whereby the body then can examine and venture out to find new and yet disregarded irregularities throughout the body and take the appropriate action to remove them. This would seem to be a major functional least associated to a degree with the liver, who as it would seem when a person eats throughout the day especially snacks into the evening, creates a situation where the liver constantly and continually works, thus never having a chance to reset, basically becoming exhausted resulting in a reduced or weakened immune systems.

Dr. Jason Fung not only discovered this factor but also

demonstrated many of the benefits that seem to be initiated, improved, or in some cases sicknesses or systemic disorders that are eliminated all by using this Intermittent Fast. It would seem by merely initiating something that appears to be associated with fasting, a plethora of gifts are received back for God, who does the healing merely because the person decides to do it, not even necessarily doing for God?

One would venture to say if a person decided to do this fasting and even did it as reason, no other than to honor God for the health they hope to receive in the body, of which God gave them as well, the multiple and seemingly endless list of potential gifts in return would speak to the essence of God not only in the fasting method but in the health atmosphere altogether.

All I know is since I started practicing this intermittent fasting, which by the way merely consists of not eating until noon, eating anything I want lunch, snacks in-between, and then dinner, to end eating about eight or so at night, not only have I stopped snoring and had much more restful sleep, but any form of allergy altogether has disappeared. The snoring thing alone was something that countless visits to the doctor and at least three operations could do nothing to help? Suddenly and almost miraculously just telling the dark spirit to leave in prayer and using this simple fast a few times was enough!

As a matter of fact over the course of the last year or so since my wife Anna insisted we start this, neither one of us has come down with anything other than a momentary sniffle and those merely lasted but an hour or two, just long enough for us to recognize them, tell them to leave and then thank God for delivering us from the attack.

"Anything you do for God is as laying your treasures up in heaven, and no good seed will go to waste."

So apparently to act on something, a storm, or attack, a bit stronger than a typical irritant, a pestering little creature or simple irritation a person must use prayer to God, and then combining it with intermittent fasting or occasional fasting, will be all the weapon a person needs to fight even legions of demonic attacks.

Just Take It?

Just take it, seems to be the call sign of the general medical environment as we know it today, whether it be by the form of the patient being told to "Take It!" being a pill, a dose of chemo, a recommended procedure that seems fruitless but needing to be done anyway, or merely the recommended direction and authorization being told to practitioners dished out with little or no explanation, and even less sympathy for the actual one needing help. People are being told to take something upon themselves, often in the form of new names defining who or what they are, using the same word we might use or interpret to mean; "just allow it" because there is nothing you can do about it, or because a so-called doctor tells you so. Just like taking a beating from a bully, waiting in pain, and producing fear until the blows subside.

Most injured people in my experience as a caregiver, generally just take it, especially when it comes to dealing with afflictions or diseases. Some might say that taking penicillin or even choosing to exercise after getting an injury is a way of fighting back, but in reality, patients are often told or even coerced to just follow like blind sheep where they are told even if the instruction is clearly over the cliff into the ocean? But I have to say that as people get older they seem to more and more resolve themselves into the notion that these processes are inevitable and they are doomed to suffer these issues eventually anyway, so the mere will to try to fight back even when it comes to a simple choice of taking medications or exercising with therapy seems like an increasing lost cause.

Our first mistake in that statement is people don't just get anything, they suffer from attacks from the outside, or worse yet open the gates of their own private temples to the attacking hordes that rush in. This is an open invitation to their bodies themselves, executed by their own actions, experiences, words, or very thoughts manifest in our creative natures through our beliefs into realizations of the world around us and within us. More than any other way they precipitate the majority of attacks by the word preceding out of their own mouths.

Jesus himself said; *"It is not what goes into the mouth but what precedeth out that corrupts a Man."*

People often just take it, because they have either been convinced that they are powerless to do anything about it, or are misguided into thinking the course of action actually will improve their lives even after they had to reduce their own life with the self-claimed new name or title. Most of the time through misconceptions of the world and who they may have become, some misconceived notion of who they are destined to be, and in some more malevolent cases; because their own suffering actually profits the one doing the telling. Nowhere have I seen more examples of this than in the highest-paid areas of health care.

The majority of the patients I have worked with over the years had a predisposed idea of the course of their illness or injury, and for the majority of them a simple resolution seemed to precipitate their expectations based initially upon whatever the doctor happens to tell them, but lately, it was more based simply on something they read on the internet than anywhere else. Basically, they give up before even trying!

Individuals in authority, with greed as the basis for their prescription lie to injured or suffering people for their own personal gains whether it be profit or worse simple evil wishing inwardly the child's utter detraction, amounts to little more than vultures who feed upon the weak.

Also, I have found that people who didn't have this predisposed course of development or lack thereof, would for the majority of the time feel that they were getting exactly what they basically deserved because of some vivid action or habit they happen to practice years even decades before?

I guess this amounts to another lie whispered into innocent ears for the purpose of doubt and despair. The soon to be conquered must first be convinced to fear! Such whispers are perpetrated by the world designed for one purpose to convince God's children that they were created less than the way He created them to be.

We are all created perfect, remembered not forgotten, sought out and not abandoned, and most importantly forgiven with the sacrifice of God's Own Son and never Unforgiven. I Am is a God that while giving every one of us of our life, has given us all the structures and support we will need to overcome all of the attacks we are meant to overcome.

Suffering through, weathering the storm, lying down, and taking the beating, or settling for continuous and unrelenting pain and even death as a possible solution to just overcome, does not take faith but relies on doubt, doubt in God for answers to the issues and the attacks at hand.

As a medical provider I can honestly say that even back in my own education decades ago we were taught to instruct patients to blindly listen to our advice, trust only the accepted licensed medical providers of the specific areas, seeing everything outside the practice pharmaceutical insurance authorized mindset as hocus-pocus even to the point of if a solution wasn't possible by us, then one doesn't exist.

For the many, the idea of merely surviving has been perpetuated into the consciousness of people, granting unto them a posture that abandons Faith and takes on an attitude of voluntary enslavement. Posture is everything, and if we have a posture of a slave we are a slave. I have seen so many people as they gain years of experience take on the very posture of the journeys they so fervently try to hide?

"This is the battle for our very soul!"

Peter Colla

Stand and Fight!

Bullies demonstrate themselves in many forms, not always limited to the pimple-faced somewhat overweight boy, large in stature for no other reason than the fact that at least one time being held back in the early stages of his education experience, gave him the illusion that he was actually bigger than others. Lacking as much in the cute existential comment department as they do in compassion, but always presenting their own hearts that drives them to particular behaviors of cruelty perpetrated against weaker defenseless opponents, bullies present oftentimes for reasons known only to their own jealous desires.

Once said bully is spotted, or at least finds himself within striking range, one of three responses for the would-be victim usually is eliminated especially if the Bully has already placed claws or filthy teeth on soft innocent flesh.

The first either, "Turn and Run," option is thwarted leaving only the "Just Take It?" or in some stronger and rarer cases "The Fight"? But first, we will further examine the run and hide option in part.

Turning represents a physical changing direction from the path in which one has been set. When a person turns their back on something, it becomes difficult, if not impossible, to see it, thus the person becomes blind to everything that lies down that particular path they were on only moments before. Not to mention turning from the path on which one has set their mind to in itself brings a notion of defeat?

Turning one's back on the attacker puts them into the victim role in a particularly vulnerable position, by presenting one's back, inviting attack without defense, blind to any blows, tail tucked in pathetic attempt to protect private parts in the backside of running retreat. Protecting private parts, now that's a statement; trying in some desperate way to protect a person's destiny, the not yet conceived future, even maybe their children, holding tightly to a hope that not only pain will be avoided, but maybe other daybreaks warmth still might be found shining on their face, if only through survival.

In the case of disease or other spontaneously occurring afflictions, many of these seem to arise without a specific physical event tied to the cause. But remember we are taught that diseases, which by the way we can never see because they are too small to see, too faint to smell, too light or few to feel, we just know or believe them to be real because we have been told they are.

But we are also programmed to feel we are absolutely helpless to these attacks, and the eventual destruction they might inflict, or at least we are told from our earliest memories. We don't see them, feel them or know for sure they are even present, but we are told, taught, and convinced they are real, the symptom in our body is the proof, and in most cases, the symptom of our body fighting them has been misconceived to be the actual sickness itself. Example; "you have a fever!" The fever is not the sickness but the result of the person's body trying to rid itself of a would-be attacker.

"Amazing how fear can make the most insignificant speck of essence into a giant."

But let us make one thing clear, we are talking about a bully here, not standing and fighting battles we are not prepared or equipped to, nor called to fight against in our proper time, by Him who would command us, is foolish. Running, and while in certain undeniable and overpowering attacks, survival can in itself find certain qualities of victory, but for the sake of the bullying, or in this case the very start of an affliction, we can assume that God will never place His children who seek Him in a place where defeat is possible unless He is calling us home. God keeps all of His promises, remember?

Avoiding the storm altogether; which includes changing the direction you are walking through this journey which is your life, is not a bad idea, especially when the direction is wrong or destructive for you or others for that matter. But changing directions is not always feasible, considering some storms come up on people so fast and unexpected, it is almost impossible to avoid them.

I have noticed people who often avoid contact with infections at all cost or take extreme almost fanatic actions to isolate themselves from injuries, they end up wallowing in fear more than not and catch the very thing they fear anyway.

When a person does happen to see the danger and chooses a different path, leaves the previous experience or issue unresolved it will result in a constant searching in the dark bushes or looking over the shoulder waiting for attack posture of fear, and a distraction from the path immediately results. Take your eye off of where you are going or where exactly you are stepping and a fall is imminent.

Fear that the bully or storm may show up along the new path taken results and this can be so overpowering that this fear actually begins to smell, the enemy can smell it. Fear is taken on by the child, like having a red cloak draped around the quivering shoulders in the middle of a field, and the angry bull is then immediately attracted to, resulting in the very thing the poor child fears. Remember what we are dealing with here, these creatures are like animals, and like animals, they can smell fear. These spirits live to be known and feed on fear! Fear is all they have, they have it and they desire it themselves, they are drawn to it as flies are to a dying carcass.

Both results running or just taking it, are not the most desirable, and often result in the child having to usually suffer the brunt of the storm anyway.

No matter how a child tries to avoid or run, it seems like the bully always seems to find us and confrontation is inevitable.

So turning and running, for the most part, demonstrates and grants if not directly, inevitably assured defeat! Nobody ever wants to feel like a coward yet the feeling is put on us by ourselves when we run from the path we thought we should be on, because of fear, this dirty feeling is inevitable.

So that leaves us one choice, yes, with bullies and diseases; the best is to stand your ground and fight.

For God has said in many places throughout the Bible; *"I will give you all you need!"*

"But my God shall supply all your need according to His riches in glory by Jesus Christ." Philippians 4:19

Also "Seek ye first the kingdom of God and His righteousness, and all things shall be given unto you." Matthew 6:33

Notice He says; *"seek ye first,"* so by assumption, if we are seeking first, doing what we are supposed to, in each and every one of our steps, then we can also assume, by His promise, that He will give us all we need to overcome any challenge, any attack that presents itself on this path?

But God also doesn't honor the footsteps of fools. If we by our own selfish desires, pride, lust, arrogance, or whatever, find ourselves not only off the path but knee-deep in the camp of the enemy, then getting everything we need to overcome, may just reside in a pair of good legs and enough oxygen in the blood to get us out of there with barely our skin.

Back to the bully, if running is defeat, it still results in two things that only a good God could even remotely turn to positive; it reduces the value, the stature of our would-be hero in the eyes of most watching, those eyes of himself being the greatest affected. Popular phrases that one will often hear include; "Once a coward always a coward," "You chicken," or "Scattering of the roaches" these just being a few of the endearing terms, that have been associated with people who flee. Gods ability to even turn this into positive is without dispute, for no other reason than just because He said so, but we will have to reserve this topic for future writing.

The second effect of running is that it builds the confidence of said bully. Making it more likely he will just do his mouthing-off again, louder next time, more often, and cause even more damage in the next or direct vicinity. So confident is the bully of where he has been that he doesn't even look back himself. And why should he, only the conquered reside behind him? But it is in his confidence that he exposes his weakness.

There is the third choice, "Stand and fight".

"Do not fear, I am with you!"

I remember as a youth running and avoiding a bully for many months and possibly as much as a year until finally, I resolved myself I would not run again. Taking my normal route home I turned around some bushes along the path home just to find myself face to face with the bully.

A larger boy with a reputation for the cruelty immediately started to advance but slowed when I held firm and said; "well I guess if we need to do this, we do?" Putting my hands up to defend myself.

Now I know the larger boy saw the fear in my eyes and his advance was certain, but the confidence quickly subsided as he looked past me at the figure who just stepped around the bushes after me. Ronny Mayberry an even larger more athletic boy from the same class suddenly steps from around the path and immediately moves towards the would-be bully taking him firmly by the collar and stating in no uncertain terms that his bullying days were over.

While there wasn't much of size a difference between them it was clear who was confident and now who was afraid. The would-be bully whimpered and made his promise and to my knowledge never bullied anyone again.

"Bullies like diseases are really cowards in disguise, turn on the light and they always run."

Ronny was an angel sent by God, he may have not even known it any more than the bully knew he was being used?

The essence of reality, funny how is it that people are so easily convinced what is reality and what is not, purely based on perspective, experience, images or sounds they have been fed, or even what others have merely told them. With medicine or in the case of sicknesses it is amazing how peoples symptoms will actually start matching the perspective symptom list of an injury the very moment the person thinks they actually have it, even if these same people never demonstrated the original symptoms in any other areas of their bodies, so strong is the mind and positive or in this case negative is its' reinforcement.

The effect of negative reinforcement, where negative suggestions or images, sounds or ideas actually are reinforced being felt or imagined symptoms. This is nowhere more evident than in health care and the people claiming understanding and knowledge, doing the telling know nothing about the where these things actually come, what prompts or motivates the diseases or even that they are motivated by something, where they are going, as a matter of fact, our entire medical health care temple with all of its potions and procedures cannot cure a single affliction or ailment, only God can.

As a matter of fact, it was a very disconcerting realization that with the exception of a few skilled individuals using techniques as old as civilizations themselves, repairing or even replacing damaged tissues with healthy undamaged replacements from others, very few procedures actually stimulate healing, but merely reduce symptoms of other injuries suffered earlier. I guess this all amounts to just taking it instead of actually fighting back.

So how do we actually fight?

"Standing and Fighting" grants and demonstrates certain victorious portions! Victory is a victory!

By definition first, a person must "Stand," that is get up, rise, now with this image carries a meaning of an immediate and direct increase in stature. When a person rises to the occasion, they grow larger, and in a direct counter, their opponent will decrease, if by no other means than just a simple vantage point. As a person being attacked gets higher, the object against which one stands appears smaller.

To stand also implies finding a firm foundation, one can only successfully achieve a firm foundation if they press against something also firm, the rock being the strongest, but make no mistake even a deep foundation in the sand, the key being deep, can be a significant pillar for resistance. God describes studying the Word as finding a deep foundation or building on the rock, both apply, but basically looking to God in any method is sufficient for the building.

As I have already stated the physical changes that one will benefit from in standing and fighting, those being first an increase of the defender, and a decrease of the attacker, is crucial for a change in momentum and status. These are immediate and Godly provisions given by the natural laws that nobody can deny. There is movement and that movement is backward into a realm the giant never looks, he has no experience there.

But let us examine further some supernatural effects, those just under the skin.

What must have gone through Goliath's mind, and maybe even that dark hole which represents his heart, when David walked out there unto the battle plane? And we might even possibly take a glance at what may have been going on supernaturally, in and around the environment.

First, in Goliath's experience, everyone who had ever faced him ran, only the poor unfortunate's that he may have been chased down, fought back in some kind of pathetic defense as he dished out his cruel blows, or just played on the ground screaming their pathetic "no waits" as he swung down his death blows from above. For an oversized opponent, the forward motion has its advantages, as any football player on the line will tell you, once you get them back on their heels you can push them anywhere. The forward momentum of any type is a force that must be resisted, held in check, overcome, and eventually overpowered in order to turn a would-be victim into any type of victorious posture. A very difficult situation when facing something that big, no maybe the largest warrior to ever step on a battlefield?

So when Goliath saw someone actually step up and faced him, even just a boy moving towards him rather than away, most likely doubt from witnessing something new and yet unseen must have at least tickled the edges of his senses, a small yet inconceivable new experience just under his skin? It wasn't tickling the hordes of the supernatural, for the wave of force that shot through their ranks most assuredly shook them to their black bones. Remember these are forces created by God and empowered by His promises, good things, real waves, Godly waves, and darkness always flees when the Light shows up.

He was bigger than anyone, so fighting from a height

advantage in downward blows, always allowed him to engage much stronger muscle groups than having to fight upward. Goliath was used to only his forward motion, using his imposing size, weight, and great strength and most importantly his "postured fearful image" to do most of his work for him.

When David stood his ground, the increased advantage, even if it had been but a slight decreasing effect on Goliath, was a decrease none-the-less! Anyone who participates in any kind of sports activity will tell you momentum is a powerful thing, and when someone starts downward or decreasing in trend, that it is usually coupled with some kind of loss and or even pain. The pain signal starts ringing, the attack is coming!

Next, David not only took Goliath's insults and threats but laughed at them and responded with his own, backed by the power of the Creator of the Universe, Reality instead of just shadows!

Oops!

Suddenly Goliath's words that usually made his opponent's quiver made this person laugh, but notice Goliath wasn't laughing, he was too busy shaking from the apparent Lion's roar he just heard! Something was seriously wrong here for

Goliath, and for the first time in his life, he might have even felt that cold chill go literally up to his spine, and if he wasn't, he should have been!

Momentum shifting, from Goliath moving forward his whole life, to being suddenly held in check, someone stepping up, him shrinking in stature, and getting less than expected result from his threats, even resulting in further diminishing on the bullies part. Momentum had now at this instant shifted! The lights were on and blazing!

Goliath threw out a desperate comment, trying to weaken David with statements of; "You come at me like a dog, with a stick." His comment was not as much of a joke, but a feeble attempt, for it was designed to make David believe he was ill-equipped to the task.

But David's faith and the trust he had everything he would need from God to defeat this man, threw the insult right back stating that Goliath's weapons were nothing compared to that of the Living God. And if Goliath's eyes weren't wide with fear at the power of these words, they were the moment the giant took but a single step forward and David started running straight towards him!

At every turn, victory was accomplished, and the actual

deliverance had not even been dealt out yet. In everyone's eyes, natural and in the supernatural, there was no doubt as to the sudden cease and immediate reversal of the momentum.

I can imagine on the barren plane of the supernatural where a horde of demonic legions stood moving comfortably forward against the children of God, riding on the backside of Goliath's image, the attack's and effect's of the constant bombardment of fear, doubt, hopelessness, rejection, abandonment, and doom, must have been nearly overpowering to the soldiers of God's army, and everyone else that had ever faced the giant.

Many a troop probably were gripped in such paralyzing oppression, that they were too busy protecting their soft underbellies in some kind of fatal self-comfort, to even pick up the sword and shield that lied only a handbreadth from them to fight back, so gripping is the fear of hopelessness. I can hardly imagine the refreshing warmth that must have flowed over the children like anointing oil on dry cracked skin, as the demon horde immediately stopped the attack, withdrawing suddenly not unlike habits running for their holes, into their own defensive positioning at the sign of the sudden and direct momentum shift exploding in front of them like a nuclear explosion of bright Holy Light!

Thousands of smaller demons squealed and ran almost immediately as the Light went on! "A Scattering of the Roaches" does apply here very nicely! There must have also been an immediate withdrawing of the more herd animal-type troops, running in every direction the spiritual screams would surely have been audible in the murmurs of the physical troops. The more seasoned and some might say powerful spiritual troops first knowing that they were going to be held accountable for the butt-kicking that was coming, may have tried to pull back hard as it was not to run, they may even try to interlock their own spiritual shields in some kind of desperate counter defensive. This had no doubt, sent that physical twinge up the spine of not only Goliath but all of the Philistine troops assembled, cold and lonely was certainly its chill. A direct opposite of the counter anointing, the refreshing warmth that thrust power and confidence into the souls and bodies of the Israeli army.

But I also know when David charged, any demons of herd animal status, the entire front lines, dropped everything and ran, even trampling those who were not as fortunate to get out of the way. That's what herd animals do when someone charges. Ripples of fear and fiery Godly retribution sent choking shivers through the remaining demonic soldiers, and this feeling was backed by the power and presence of the

God who created the universe. It was a domino effect of epic proportions.

The Stone, the hurdling of the rock, the spoken manifestation, the small representation of the word of God, even in its simplest form, was all it took to open the floodgates of God's deliverance. David could have thrown anything, the giant was already doomed, but throwing out a single small piece of the Word was all it took.

Once contact was made the result was immediate and Goliath's fate was sealed. Down onto his face, Goliath fell, back exposed, demons of all ranks were running for their lives, very much emulated in the natural as the armies of the Philistine who also broke rank and ran.

At this point, all that remained was the mopping up! David casually walks up and takes Goliath's head, his victory prize to present to the king. The armies of the Living God pursue now in frenzied strength, I am sure empowered by the angelic horde that wraps themselves in and around all of the arms and souls of the Lord's army until all of the opposing force has been hunted down and killed. The Bible speaks of bodies being scattered across the countryside. It took a little time, and effort, but the victory was granted before long before the army was completely destroyed.

"Pick up your mat and walk!" How must that have sounded to the man who was himself crippled his whole life? For just a moment, wouldn't you think something dark may have whispered into his ear; "What is he crazy, you can't, you tried so many times"? Maybe he even reached up for help, but God gave him all he needed to overcome, a gentle hand and he stood?

How long after, maybe every time after he walked, and stepped just this way or that, did a feeling, a twinge in his newly healed legs, brought back a voice of the enemies whispers; "It's back, you see, temporary, a lie, you weren't really healed,"

The continuing of believing, the sharing the healing with others, that's what's called work.

The Bible tells us in John 9: 13-34, of a blind man who was cured by Jesus, and when he presented himself to the priests they tried to discredit Jesus, thus discrediting the man's healing itself, but he refused to buckle. The man stood on faith, even unto pressure, fear, ridicule, for himself, and his parents who also had been held, he held to the healing in faith, and many times confessed with his mouth; "For before

I was blind, and now I can see," "if This Man where not of God, He could do nothing."

If one could look into the supernatural at such a moment one might see such a sight;

On the barren plain, fear of the pure power of the Living God exploded through the demonic horde as fast as a blast of irradiated light of the greatest flash ever witnessed. The front line buckles and explodes in a moment. From a barrier and confidence that has been no doubt built over years, toppled in a moment. As the demonic troop scatters, a wall of dark black bricks is clearly seen, most likely that of which these creatures have been leaning against, hiding, almost secretly building inside the courtyard of God's beautiful child's eyes for years?

He takes a hand full of the arrows, yet unused, some that have yet to hit their intended mark, and he throws them down in a thunderous explosion. "From the ground you come and into the ground you shall go again!" "If This Man were not of God, He could do nothing."

The ripple of the power sends a shock wave through the ground like a massive earthquake wave right into the enemies camp, and like a vast wave rolling through a calm still black lake, so confident they were in their hold and position there wasn't even a ripple on the surface of their dark waters, until now.

As the wave explodes through the dark waters, it becomes clear and sure to see, not deep were their murky secrets, an illusion of lies and deceit. The wave gathers strength as it approaches the wall, it seems to be powered by his momentum, and that of the Word, exploding into the dark wall sending it toppling like a flimsy card house of black dominoes.

Facedown in the muck lies the one that yelled; "How dare you tell me I can see, it's not my time yet!"

The worm-faced giant lay face down in the muck, back exposed waiting only for death's victory to be dealt out.

The recently blind but now victoriously seeing child stamps the shadows mercilessly into the ground with mere words, for they showed him no mercy as they tried to steal his gifts.

Time to mop up! He stamps the image of sickness into the ground in defiance.

Yes, there are groups of fleeing troops that have run to the trees, waiting for some reinforcements for small counterattacks. Waiting for orders, they still turn and fling their arrows of doubts. Tossing accusations against those who helped him, doubt, challenges to him to turn and run, more doubt, calling to him "if you doubt any you must doubt all," trying to shake even his faith that God could or would help him, more doubt, but now his shield is up and deflection is becoming something he is beginning to master. One by one each of these little attacks fall, time, distance, and perseverance must follow to mop up the entire army.

Victory is undeniable! The stronghold has been toppled! Now the mess has to be cleaned up, many dirty bricks lay around, held together in the memories of mortar and ash. The black ash water is just settling, the clear water pressing the ash into the soil soon to become the fertilizer of another beautiful patch of garden. His house, his lands are called to be a garden, not a barren plain of ash and dark.

Yes, there will be skirmishes, troops will attack, some he may lose, but many he will win, and ever will their numbers slowly dissipate until the last of the retreating horde finds itself defeated or banished. On he goes to tell others of the gift he has been given, a gift of love and light, a free gift, a promised gift.

So is it.

"Dear Lord please open my eyes, those of my friends, and my loved ones, to the lies of the enemy, give us strength, wisdom, and discernment as to Your path for our lives, and the battles You would have us fight."

"Amen"

Light VS Dark

The world would have us believe the opposite is true. People get a concussion, in the dark, they go, get a cut or wound in the dark with bandaging, even desire to know more about the process you may be suffering from, nothing, you are in the dark about it! Throughout my career, I have been often told to render my belief, not to my own understanding or feelings, but as in the case of sicknesses or injuries defer the determination and outcomes to others who have been given authority and are declared experts, merely because they have attended a few classrooms of instruction or received authorization from some factor that seems to be in charge, unknown, aloof, and resting just above the realm of understanding, I or we have been given. Seems spiritual to me?

I have even seen recently, even in areas where I was declared an authority or expert, even in these cases the authorization to treat in this way or that, to be granted it would have to first be run by one of final determination often for costs, participation, or effectiveness in collaboration, basically by an insurance company, of which they now have to approve of providers, as it was credentialing them, even long after training is completed or certifications given by the state governing bodies.

What was funny as I began to question the entities making the decisions, I found more often than not, the people making the decision regarding a particular person's healthcare directions had little if any formal training, and merely based the decision on a set guideline being declared by the assigned diagnosis code? For those who don't know what a diagnosis code is, today every sickness, or injury, affliction or anything that has to do with healthcare must be assigned a diagnosis code. This code then comes with an exact definition that must be applied to the person who is requesting treatment. In fact, any variation whatsoever from the accepted and recommended course of action was not only discouraged but in many cases followed by a threat of exclusion for both the person receiving care and the provider!

The system as it stands has, in essence, takes away all aspects of faith and places a sense of absolutism into the hands of the very people or spirits who merely wish to control and enslave you into an ideology of complete submission, doubt, and hopelessness. This I am sure is by design as these institutions that use fear and confusion to manipulate and then enslave children who have given themselves over to the authority of this belief.

I have heard it commonly said that; "The monetary systems of the world" are not persons but a temple, a temple where we are manipulated to put our faith in, and later our prayers, finally our entire devotion and sacrifices.

The current medical model as it has developed into, is also a temple, and if it is by definition or even essence a temple, then it must have a dark spirit behind it, who wishes to be a god at least as it pertains to us. With a dark agenda, it cannot be anything but dark itself, with a purpose that has no other desire than to entangle, enslave, and be worshiped as a god.

The temple then sets out to educate its experts like priests and priestesses, or servants in a very narrow-minded view of what and how it would describe its particular area of God's creation that it wishes to steal for itself, in this particular case; the assurance of health and healing. They cannot operate themselves for they are but spirits, and need physical beings to do their dirty work, the top spokesmen or women, high priests, and priestesses, the ones who can do the most damage or lever the most influence would have the greatest treasures rained upon them. While they may think they even receive power, yet know this, as the slave masters of old, they are also slaves themselves, for they will never be the true masters for these are dark malevolent spirits, and as slaves, the servants must only do what they are told, when they are told, no matter how many people they know will be harmed?

The spirit seduces its believers first with the promise of success, wealth, and health, but eventual strives towards domination, control, and dependency to ensure everybody must come to them, and only them, for this specific slice of God's creation of which He intended for every one of us, that is this institution's mark, this temples deep lust in its attempts to steal from us.

This is done by restricting access to healing only through the use of its priests, its doctors, its educators, it tells them how and when they must treat, and limits them in the means or agents they may use to treat, levying incomprehensible cost on anyone who wishes to use its services, to place access out of the normal hands of it future servants. And if the doctors see the truth and try to stand against it, the temple will just expel them from participation, destroy them, or even kill them, if they try to deviate out of the recommended course of action.

It uses darkness to treat darkness, threats, and fear to elicit belief in its victims, only occasionally throwing a crumb to a starving dog, which merely has the effect of giving the person treating, a momentary satisfaction from the burden they are addressing, merely to become a pawn for future payments. This is done one spoon at a time, "Orphans Porridge" in effect, and is a cleaver sowing of weeds into a perfect garden attempt to slowly build more toxins and poisonings in God's children, that over time, eventually becoming more dependent and enslaved in the system. This dark spirit has no interest in curing anything, merely hooking all the fish in the pond and slowly pulling them in until they are all hooked on whatever pill they happen to have a weakness for.

This temple, this assurance, it is a place that wishes your full prayers and devotion, your first fruits, and eventually even the sacrifice of your very children.

The masses are brainwashed in believing that they were created with flaws and destined to acquire the very issues they trying to avoid with the drugs they are taking. They are taught from the earliest age that sicknesses are something they are predestined to, or inherit from their parents, and all they can do is sit back and hope, maybe pray, that the big bad sickness monster doesn't come to visit them while they sleep. People are taught they are insignificant, constantly evolving, thus insufficient, weak, and vulnerable to the smallest of creatures, these fiendish entities always lurking ready to pounce on innocent flesh at any moment. While part of this is true, the part about the sicknesses being the smallest of creatures waiting to pounce on command, but the part that is not true is that we are weak, evolving, insignificant, and vulnerable to them.

This goes exactly against the Word of God which talks about us being special and significant, being created perfect, being strong, and able to overcome all adversity. "I chose to believe what God says rather than what the world says." He also said He knew every one of us even before He created the known universe, so how could we possibly be evolving? We are not we are growing, growing with the continual and new experiences of God's gifts daily in our lives.

As a result, the masses sit and fear, as they are being told there is nothing they can do about it, no amount of exercise or healthy eating can stop it if you are destined to get it, or so they are told. So keep going to the doctor with any symptoms or inkling, so the doctor can get you on a regimen of drugs to stop the issue before it gets too bad to handle. I have even seen today advertisements for cancer medications whereby people are promoted to take prior to getting cancer.

We are told to "Fear Not," yet fear is enveloped into every advertisement, every test, every consultation a person participates with? Fear that a person might have this or that, and consequently cause them to either lose what functions, or the very life they already have, or fail to heal and regain what they may have already lost, if a particular regiment of obedient "Just take it" is not followed. What gets me is the long list of possible side effects the pharmaceutical companies must list as a disclaimer tool, hopefully freeing themselves from being sued if a person decides to take the drug? The side effects are often so much more dilapidating than the original issue the person was trying to receive assistance with.

Once we are willing to look at health care and thus our own sicknesses from a more spirit-minded approach, then perhaps we will take one step further and apply this spiritual application to sicknesses and the treatments of these?

Let's try it!

The First Simple Step in Healing Yourself; Don't Believe The Lies, and thus believe there is possibly more of a spiritual side to healthcare than you have been told? Just in that moment of belief is the switch for turning on the light, actually turned on!

When I first began to examine the possibility that a more supernatural occurrence may be in play in the area of healing, I placed into me as a practitioner in an immediate and almost perplexing notion; "Why do some people get healed and others seem to not?"

I have seen it played out time and time again, whereby people with seemingly the exact issues and the exact condition, one will recover and sometimes even in miraculous manners, while others seem to have their issue continue with seemingly no long-term elevation, no matter what is done?

At first glance the issue could be attested to the age or condition of the person being treated, perhaps it is pre-disposition or their nutritional habits, maybe it is other habits that hinder or stimulate such rapid recoveries or lack thereof? But the more I seemed to delve into studying the patterns of recovery and the greater the cases quantities that were examined the sooner I realized that no set factors or relative principles could be determined that would attest to one specific advantage or not, other than the obvious age-related advantages, and even these often would from time to time present also anomalies that defied explanation; such as young children who would not recover even with seemingly minimal pertinent afflictions, while some elderly also would almost miraculously recover with only the simplest and brief interventions.

I immediately began to examine various aspects of healing and how these related to manifested particularities of what people associated with, or referred to as miraculous healings. Examining aspects of prayer and what effect this had on patients knowing or even unknowingly engaged. Various aspects of natural medicines were increasingly used in the therapeutic venue also to attempt to see if by inclusion any of these or possibly all of them may lead to increased effectiveness of the treatment regiments already considered.

In essence, I was searching for the key to discovering what I referred too and I may understand it as the "God Gene". It was a blind adventure that lasted months even years, as various aspects of the natural were presented, tried, and tabulated always adding these procedures into the already present model.

The result; when I added anything that was natural, good, loving, or Godly, people would have positive results, many instantaneous and completely unexpected. But I found that with many the results didn't last. People would return days, weeks, or even moments later with a return of the same symptoms.

Over time I began to realize that this is because we were only treating a fraction of the person, touching upon the symptoms, great or small, these are only the smallest fraction of the actual story that represents every person that presents themselves for treatment.

If you want to fix a broken house, and all you do is fill a single crack on the wall with a little plaster and paint, you are doomed to not only have a very small success rate, you are actually guilty of inadvertently being paid for nothing.

I not so quickly, I must shamefully admit, realized that if you want to heal people with a large amount of success you must treat the whole person, thus examine the entire person. But what was exactly the entire person? We are more than just bodies, feet, knees, backs, ligaments, muscles, skin, systems, blood, brains, hearts, or pieces. We are more than just minds, with experiences past, present, and even dreamed about in the future. We are more than just beliefs with every emotion, hope, love, desire, hate, aspiration, and fear. We are an accumulation of all of these things.

So knowing this, how does a person who wants to effectively help another person heal and desires to affect this healing on all levels, as to increase the effectiveness of said treatment, how does a person examine the issues on all these levels simultaneously?

I had no idea so I asked.

"You start by turning on the light."

"Turning on the light is nothing more than asking God what is going on?"

"You have not because you ask not. And ask anything in My name and I will grant you even more than I had done on earth because I am in heaven with My Father."

"Again Promises!"

Step one Ask God. Turn on the light, lift your head, just like with Michelle, call out and whatever God reveals, act on it.

"Just being willing to look in the direction of God is the first act of faith."

I immediately went on a program during the examination to have people not only tell me what happened physically to them when they first felt the injury or affliction but what exactly were they busy within their minds at the time of the attack and more importantly what they were struggling within in their belief systems, what was pulling at them at that particular time in their lives?

What was amazing was the injury almost every time mimicked in the location of attack issues they were struggling with their bodies, their very souls, for example, people who were carrying heavy burdens in their family might suddenly sustain a back issue, people struggling with the direction they may be going in a career, a hip or knee, people who hold onto emotions weight issues, people having problems letting go intestinal, the list goes on and on?

People with great issues of carrying burdens in their life resulting in compounded issues in their back, would state that virtually all of them at the moment of the injury they would remember that they may have been struggling with thoughts or worrying concerns of such issues? People who were having issues deciding which direction to go might develop neck problems, especially when times of great concerns or distractions precipitated. Shoulders for issues of great mobility or lack thereof in their current situations. Heart problems for people struggling with family issues or decisions they had made that affected their families. Intestinal problems with people having a hard time letting go of the past issues, weight problems when they would stuff emotionally, cancer when battles would rage within them. But what then what to do about it?

Amazingly, though the correlation of spiritual significance a comparison occurred to a like physical location? What does this mean? Is it important? Another thing to turn the light on about I guess?

Anxiety with unresolved fears, balance when the confusion of their life became unbearable and unresolvable. Lung problems with people who had issues with speech, eye problems when they knew they were looking in the wrong places. On and on the similarities emerged and frankly what was amazing was that in every case when people were willing to examine that there might be a spiritual meaning to the event or attack in their life, they almost always and completely knew exactly what and why it was happening to them and the organs or extremities involved. A sort of Godly awareness would occur, Godly wisdom for those who ask.

So the solution seemed obvious after you turn on the light the next step is to just simply and quietly ask why?

Why this issue, at this time, in this place on my body? What are you supposed to learn from this experience, remember what doesn't kill you makes you stronger? God can turn all things to good for those who seek Him.

What are you supposed to learn at the moment of the attack, what are you to overcome? How are you to be better, stronger, wiser, it is at this moment of asking the lights come on, wisdom appears, and the darkness must flee?

What Doesn't Kill Us Makes Us Stronger

But for those who happen to survive the storms, is granted another promise; What doesn't kill you makes you stronger.

In health care this statement while I have heard it said my entire life seems to be the hardest to comprehend. In some cases, people are born with issues, or later have such dilapidating injuries, illnesses, or accidents they seem to never get better or if they survive they seem to suffer, leaving the observer with a perplexing realization that the statement what doesn't kill us makes us stronger just doesn't apply to these?

It really does, it applies to everyone that survives, what doesn't kill you makes you stronger is not just a statement to boost morale, but an inevitable truth that merely needs to be realized. People survive and become greater in themselves or better, but in many cases delve only on to that which is lost rather than looking at the miracle of healing and the realization of the gift of getting stronger the survival realizes. This is a truth, and truths are rained down on everyone's heads as indiscriminately as rain upon all the children's heads equally and freely, another promise, one and the same!

I started to think if there was ever an example of anyone I may have treated that one might think didn't get stronger?

I have personally treated many examples of people who either have lost limbs, gone blind, ruptured disks or just people who have suffered from sicknesses especially brutal ones such as cancer who while they seem to get a little better, a fraction may be through relief of pain doesn't seem to ever get better than they were before, most worse, yet the most dramatic case that comes to mind was when I first started treating the case of JW?

Suddenly a flash of memories of a person I hadn't treated or thought of in nearly twenty-five years came back to mind as clear as it were yesterday, and this is what I remember about JW.

I remember early in my career a man by the name of JW, and while that is not his name, I have no idea how I might find him, if he is still alive to ask him permission to speak about my experience with him, so I will change the name, as I do with every example of real people I write about, to protect their privacy.

One day JW rolled into my office being pushed in his wheelchair. He was severely disfigured, having nearly half of his body ripped off in a heavy construction accident, he presented himself as a mere part of a person, torn, in pain, and angry.

As the story goes JW was in charge of manning the end of an enormous digger on the end of a conveyor belt-like machine having multiple digging buckets clawing into the ground as massive amounts of earth were dug away and then displaced along in a conveyor-like manor back bchind the larger machine behind, to later be picked up by other large loading machines and carted off for processing in whatever extraction this machine was designed to fulfill?

JW expressed that there was a fail-safe at the end of the machine that would override the controller sitting back in the cab of the almost house size machine so that if he was in trouble the machine would immediately shut down. But on many occasions, this shut-off would be defective, and because of the great amount of debris and dust kicked in the air it was impossible for the controller up in the cab to see the front-man all the time.

On this particular day, as much as he could remember, a

large stone was ripped from the ground under where he stood and he fell in with one leg having his boot become caught by the teeth of the large digging claw, dragging him into the machine and ground.

He woke up moments later being rushed to the hospital, died at least five and maybe seven times on the operating table just to finally be saved as finding himself now in this wheelchair for life.

The claw must have pulled down onto his right shoulder because nearly half of his body was gone. His right shoulder, half of his right side of his chest, his whole right hip, and below were gone. His left leg was severed halfway across the middle of the thigh, all of which left this poor man disfigured, and with severe scoliosis not able to sit straight in any practical chair.

But that wasn't all, his face was maimed to the point where he had lost half of his jaw, one of his two eyes, and literally, a part of his face and skull leaving him disfigured to the point where it was amazing he could even be alive.

He told us he wanted to have treatment for the pain, suffering from pain every day and constant. We treated him for a while, and being nearly twenty-five years ago I don't remember much about him or whether or not he had gotten any better, I do remember he came in for a while, received a fairly large settlement from the accident, and had the same caregiver always come in with him, a pleasant lady who never left his side.

I do also remember being intrigued with the various stories of his multiple times he died, of which he would share them with me in detail. One particular time, sharing that he had on each occasion died raised out of his body and looked down at the scene of the operating table, hearing the conversations, even knowing when the doctors would speak about giving up and allowing him to just put out of his misery, or scolding a nurse for making a rude joke during the procedure.

On one occasion he spoke about clearly lifting out of the multiple floors of the hospital and then seeing a man being moved out of a helicopter on the roof. He later told the doctor, even reporting on exactly what the man was wearing and how he had a head wound when arriving.

JW would occasionally speak of the light, and the tunnel experience, seeming to have very little memory of this and if he did wasn't sharing further details with me. This particular detail I had the most interest in at the time.

He is a good example and if; what doesn't kill you makes you stronger, how could he possibly ever have been stronger?

The part I did not realize about JW back when I worked on him, yet seem to realize now were some specific details that seemed to come to my memory all these years later, especially about the attack right at the moment of his injury. JW was divorced and had not seen his children for years struggling with the guilt and pain of this separation. On the day of his injury, he struggled with thoughts of regret and un-forgiveness for them, un-forgiveness mainly for himself.

The woman I saw who pushed him into our office was the same woman who cared for him right after his injury, and without knowing how I knew, I just did; she fell in love with him and eventually even married him.

JW was half of a man before his injury having his wife and children ripped from him, but after the injury he became a whole man again, having love and the union of man and wife in his life. He may have had half a physical body, but in his mind and more importantly in his spirit, he was a whole man again, much greater than he may have ever been before.

He shared his story with me and dozens of others, inspiring

through his suffering, yet testifying to the true healing nature of God. JW used his body now to inspire, challenge, even confront people in their deepest fears, the fragile nature of this life.

As with JW and others like him whether they are involved in accidents, injuries even of their own misguided steps, storms brought unto them merely by being in the wrong place at the wrong time, or delivered to them one spoon at a time like baby food from the spoon of a misinformed mother, the result is all the same; if you survive the ordeal, you become stronger, in spirit, mind, and even body?

Peter Colla

You Have Not Because You Ask Not

When dealing with storms in our life, God gives you everything you need to overcome any challenge, you merely have to look, reach out and take what He has already given you to overcome.

Back to the statement of; "What doesn't kill us makes us stronger" seems to find itself the least applicable in the annals of medicine, especially among health care providers, maybe it is because of the way we are taught, maybe it is because of being a first-hand witness to so many health care tragedies, but most likely it is because as any health care provider might tell you if they are honest enough to dare, is the procedures and practices that we are instructed to give really do little to actually facilitate the actual healing process. Some perhaps may help it along, but this is still a disquieting realization, that people who are long enough in the field realize, they realize that they have little if any actual effect on the healing process and it is completely and ultimately in the hands of a Higher Power, recognized by the majority of us as God.

While it is a common statement throughout the world and generally believed with only the slightest resistance, especially when people as a whole understand this statement and its application to the body as well as our life as a whole, as a medical provider especially in the past, I would probably be more on the opposite side of the fence stating when it comes to medical issues, sicknesses, especially tragic cases of injuries afflicting large parts of the body or multiple systems, the opposite is more often true, what doesn't kill us often leaves us so dilapidated, we wish we were dead.

But I am here to tell you, it is my experience after treating for decades, what doesn't actually kill them at the time of the injury, does lead to making them stronger one hundred percent of the time.

A person might say; "Well what about when a person loses a leg, what then? How are they possibly stronger?"

It doesn't matter what you think you lose, that kind of thinking especially when it comes to functions of the body, is equivalent to concentrating on what you do not have, rather than looking at what you do. Living in the past, dwelling on what you have lost, or looking at what you don't have basically is the same as staring at the shadows, or worrying about a lock of hair that you just cut.

"When you start looking at what is, rather than what is not you will find everything you need is right in front of you."

Let me tell you about Todd, as he comes to mind and I contemplate this topic.

I had a friend his name was Todd, larger than life, he was an ex-professional athlete, in his prime over six foot six, well over two hundred and eighty pounds of muscle, power, and arrogant grit. You would have to be if you wanted to play professional sports, especially in a profession where everyone is trying to throw you on your back, humiliate you, and step over you as they push forward toward their own goals. Which seems, more often than not, to have to go right through you to get where they want to go!

Todd suffered from a severe form of diabetes which he had no problem admitting or stating was his own fault, and by not taking care of his own body all those years of college even later in professional sports. Too much of everything, most of which he knew was not good for him at the time and later now seemed to cost him dearly. Todd slowly lost first the feeling in his feet, only later to begin to lose circulation in first the toes, and then progressively up until it resulted in him having to have both legs amputated in multiple and ever increasingly frequent surgeries to eventually lose both legs well above both knees.

One day he rolls in his athletic wheelchair with two temporary prosthetic legs strapped to the back, carrying a prescription to learn to walk with the legs. He was a good friend and it had been a while since I saw him so I enthusiastically said to him; "So are we going to learn how to use your legs?"

He said with angry dismay; "No! Those things are not my legs, I lost my legs, I came here to see if you could help me with this pain that will not stop killing me, and it's right there!" As he pointed to the foot peddle out in front of the chair where his foot should have been. Phantom pain, which is a pain that seems to exist in a place or extremity that is gone, was quite common with amputations, but no matter what we did for his remaining leg or his back to calm the nerve pain, nothing seemed to help.

At that time we had the son of my own martial arts instructor, John working for us as a student assistant. A 3rd-degree black-belt himself, so I thought it would at least be fun for Todd to work with him, and he quickly took a liking to the boy, Todd not thinking much of martial arts, and often saying only girls used their feet to fight. Todd would sit there and playfully try to slap at John who had no problem blocking or dodging the various almost comical antics the larger man threw at him. This relationship went on for about a week or maybe two before Todd stopped coming in.

Later John finally told me about a month or so after that Todd found it so interesting the ability to defend himself from a chair John displayed, as well as being completely surprised to hear there were entire areas of martial arts instruction that did nothing more than teach a person how to defend themselves from a chair. Todd started showing up at John's father's studio where they would roll his wheelchair out onto the mats and teach him chair-bound martial arts! Todd loved it so much he came in three to four times a week regularly now.

"That's great," I said and didn't think anything more about it until Todd walked in the office three or four months later, walking on his prosthetics, no crutches, no cane!

"Todd! My God" I said, "You look great! Who taught you to walk so fast?" He walked in and sat down in a chair in front of me, a smile on his face, and didn't say a word until I sat down myself in front facing him. At the moment I sat, my own foot slid out slightly and accidentally kicked his prosthetic leg.

"Why did you kick my leg?" He said

I never answered him, I was interested in how good he looked. The significance of his question to me I would not understand until only recently in my career, years later.

"I want to thank you." Todd said with a smile and went on, "I was here before I lost my legs," as he held out his arm at about stomach height.

"After I lost my legs, I was here!" As he put his hand down nearly to the ground holding it down there. "I was down, low, and ready to just about give it up."

"But then I started studying martial arts with John, and went there." As he raised his hand high above his head and held it there. "When I began to study the Martial Arts, walking (as he lowered his hand back to the place it was to start with) didn't seem like such a difficult thing to do anymore."

For years to come, I used Todd's story to emphasize the significance of doing something greater than the task being prescribed as a means to accomplish it; like a person learning to walk by learning to dance, or someone learning the balance of back muscles by studying Tai-Chi. But the most significant moment of the story eluded me until just recently.

When Todd first came in he said; "I'm not wearing those things, they are not my legs I lost my legs." Now he said; "Why did you kick my leg"? He got his legs back and in the process became a Martial Artist. Todd would later go on to do many things he had never done earlier, skiing, parachuting, diving, all things gained in his newfound desire to venture out and conquer since he alreacy had become a conqueror.

"Todd was a great man with a great calling, he walked through life perhaps walking the wrong direction, lost his legs, but found them again, and through this experience, he became a conqueror and now he flies."

The why, is still so difficult to stomach, and sometimes it is easy to see why some people would actually want to die than go on?

Many people long for death well before the peacefulness of it is granted, some people even understand the essentialness of results, these being an accumulation of actions all the paths and adventurers along the way it may bring. When a young person who longs for just another bright day is suddenly faced with the realization of tragic and definite dreams incomplete, it seems to often be received with a tear.

The perplexity of understanding the complexities of the failures of the body, or the reasons one or another is faced with sudden and inescapable life-ending tragedy requires an understanding that transcends the ability to understand granted in the limitations of this life.

"For now the question on the table; You have not because you ask not?"

"You have not, because you ask not, and you ask not, because you chose not to look for the answers that grant you wisdom in the direction in which it was designed to demonstrate."

Jesus demonstrated immediately and purely for those who looked to God, just by looking that direction, in a path, or eye, or ear, and even just in touch, simple rain fell in the form of healing upon every one of their heads freely regardless of their histories, races, or even religions.

All anyone had to do was, is, and will always be but ask?

Look to towards Him, if even but a touch of the hem of His garment and they know they would receive healing.

First people have to pull their own heads out from under the veils of the lies and deceits of the world, the accumulation of a lifelong series of programming, misguided teaching, and spoon-fed poisoning to even contemplate something might actually be different than we have been told. I guess death is the finish line moment of when life is complete or not?

If your race is over then you will not be able to overcome, but if you merely are to survive the ordeal and live to another day, then by definition healing has already occurred, it is you that realizes the truth within the image of your experience, then decides what to do about the messes the storms make.

If God makes you a promise, you can count on it, you can bank on it, you can bet your life on it, you can bet the farm, all wonderful terms you yourselves have created to add solid perspective to promises carved in stone, created and everlasting by Him.

God has often said life is everlasting, science says energy is everlasting, and if both are merely reflections of each other then one could believe that death is merely a consequence of turning away from God, like another stone in our garden.

They, these side-stepping jagged stones are merely momentary places we rest our feet upon as we step through the everlasting path of your soul.

Promises made, promises fulfilled, God shows us this with the appearance of signs if we but take a moment to stop and look. The promises of the rainbows, listen to the birds for they are God's messengers in Earthly form instructed to bring messages of hope and peace to those who would but stop and listen, raindrops on the faces of all His children, a gentle reminder of the free waters He gives to everyone who but lookup. The perfect individual snowflakes with their winters cold crystallized into perfected realizations that every single one is different and specifically made for each of us.

"You want to be healed, look up and ask."

Why the Leg

There is more to the story here. Why the leg?

If it is all a challenge, a task, an opportunity to overcome and grow, and if the Father can turn all things to good, then we must have a reason why the leg? The legs propel us through this life, so an attack against the legs is an attack against the very journey we find ourselves on?

So, for people who have injuries to their legs, this is an attempt to challenge their journey?

It has become evident that the reason why people would find, regarding the specifics of the attacks, these are as individual as the many individuals I would talk to? Sometimes, yes they are on the wrong path, or merely find themselves walking in the wrong direction, but sometimes they are on the right path and the challenge seems to be designed to stop them? Only each individual can come to know, and then, if they chose, overcome. Of course, this only applies to adults, children seem to have things happen to them regardless if they precipitate it themselves, that is atlas until they come to the age of accountability, are out of their control to avoid and even in some cases overcome.

So what about children, what happens when they are attacked with injuries or sicknesses?

Children are so often the intended victims of malevolent attacks, but how they react is not up to them but their parents, doctors, teachers, coaches, and other people who have been given responsibility for these innocents. In the majority of afflictions, it is the parent who needs the treatment, and through the parent the child overcomes.

Sicknesses can be fed to a child one spoonful at a time as easy as telling the same child they are sick or are something less than how they were created to be, and that is perfect.

I had personally treated children who were born with Palsy from birth, especially early in my career and it was so difficult to see perfection, and look past such drastic injuries?

But at the time I was still looking at these children through the veils of the world, not everyone is born with every blessing of the garden, the poor will always be with you, but every soul is perfect when it is created, they each get to choose light or dark in their own time when they are meant to. Hurdles are present some in obvious physical form, others with extreme mental or spiritual challenges they must face as they progress down this path we call life.

"God would that you all come to me as children, accepting the truth as the truth, unveiled and free of the shadows of earthly doubt."

Attacks against the body are storms designed to change the course of your soul through the gardens God has destined each of us individually to walk. The "why" is always present in the attack, given to us as signs to show everyone the information as to what we may learn from these experiences. This is perhaps what God meant when He said; "Be of good cheer when you are persecuted...," because knowing we will come out better and stronger can to a degree give one comfort when the pain, storm, or anguish is upon us.

In the case of legs, people who may be destined to travel great distances and do great things with the product of their steps, the enemy can't know their future nor even the essentials of what exactly this path means, the dark spirit merely sees in the supernatural a talent in the area of journey expressed in the product of manifestation that presents itself as strong legs supernaturally. So he attacks the legs as a hope to first stop the ability to journey and perhaps destroy a persons' essence of their soul the very dreams causing them to despair and give up.

How can we know if we are being attacked or on the wrong path?

Since these challenges and injuries are always attacks, we merely must go back to the source and try to surmise the essence of what is happening, where you came from, and where you are going to understand if the chosen path truly is the one? Seek knowledge from the very source of Creation, one must stop, rest, meditate or pray, and understand. If we are on a path that we know to be good and true, then the only assumption we can make is that it's an attempt to stop us.

How do you know? You will know when you are at peace.

People have a distinct understanding even genuine knowing of when they are going in the right direction and when they are not. If you are ever in doubt all you have to do is ask the One who truly is interested in your happiness?

This concept began to make so much sense, the more I began to put it into reference with the healthcare model and apply it to my own attempts at physical therapy treatments. A person who has strong legs spiritually and is destined to go to great places might be attacked in the knees stopping this motion, and at the very least has the effect of placing fear in the mind of this person in the future, preventing them from pursuing a purpose or course of their life that might involve a great deal of motion of the legs. One attack left unresolved puts fear in every thought regarding movement or travel, and thus the person allows fear to be an open window in their spiritual house in which attacking spirits can constantly revisit throughout their lives.

It is no wonder why many people will have one issue resolved may be operated on such as a ruptured disc in the back, just to have other later seemingly out of the blue rupture, without any trauma even close to the original injury.

Leave the window open the raccoons just come back later.

"Wisdom is the greatest thing you can ask for, no more so than in healing. Ask and ye shall receive!"

We were all created to lie down in green pastures and lay beside still waters, just like it says in the most famous psalm? This means basically this world was created for us to rest and enjoy without strife and in peace, but unfortunately, men have re-created a world where this has become increasingly more difficult to realize.

But for now and in this little piece of the world each of us calls our own life we can take charge and say no to attacks, claim our own piece of green grass, and lay down.

The Still Soft Voice

The very moment you feel the attack, whatever the feeling is, if it is something out of the ordinary and you feel it is negative intention against you, that is the moment of the infirmities attack and you turn the light on by becoming aware of what it really is; "tell it to leave!", basically has the effect of placing Godly intention or light directly into the issue or scene in the spirit and thus flushing out the darkness.

The very act of creating sound, positive sound, perpetuates good into the physical universe. Something new is there now that has never been there before in our present universe? It is a word that has confidence granted by God, and perpetuated with the faith that it is true and right, all these sound good to me? So by definition, if these words are a representation of light, God, faith, love, or anything positive, then they must be from the family of light, and subsequently will cause darkness to flee?

Even asking out loud for answers, the why, what lessons, which meaning, they are all the same? This too, falls in the lines of asking in faith, looking to God, praying, more light, more fleeing darkness, positive reinforcement, positive attraction, meditations, empowering, call it what you like it is all good?

Did God not say in John 14:12-14 "You will do all the things you see me do and greater because I am with my Father in heaven." The instruction is simple, just believe and ask. God has already given us authority over those dark attacking spirits. Anything we saw the greatest healer of all time demonstrate, He, Himself said we could do, and more, that being said the only thing holding us back is ourselves.

Every patient that I had ever spoken to regardless of the disease, injury, or process knew the exact moment they started feeling something wasn't right on their body, and it usually started with a little irritation or a simple pain, cough, dizziness, anxiety, cramp, stiffness, numbness, some kind of irritant that felt out of the ordinary, enough to bring their attention to it.

So why not just tell something to leave, or for that matter "command" the issue to leave the moment of the awareness before any damage can be received in our own belief? I began to talk to the people about what I was attempting myself in treatment, even going so far as to ask if they felt anything different, and then describe it, or to outright tell them I was in a sense praying for them when laying of hands was on them, this all seemed like the right approach to facilitate the God Gene into action?

As I have already said the reception was for the most part much nicer and more well-received than I had expected. Over the course of my education, the teaching community would almost with fanatic zeal infused into the minds of its students with the need to clearly and emphatically keep the ideas of God or any kind of religion out of the medical treatment arena. There was almost a sort of "Separation of Church and State" attitude placed into the health care education basis, we practitioners being the state, and while it wasn't exactly forbidden, a sense of if you did pray for your patients, don't let them know, or certainly don't tell the Doctors, unless you wanted to be blackballed as a heretic or something? But even this, when I did speak these interests and observations with colleagues, doctors, I found more than often a positive and even encouraging attitude. It was only when this method was implemented into a corporate environment, even when desired by the owner of said company, quickly certain hidden entities within certain established power levels would work diligently to destroy this application or method, and if this didn't work drive me from the company at all costs.

The people themselves, in most cases, seemed to actually be thankful for your intention to actually ask God to help them or at least a deep desire to give them something more than just the cold and unfeeling application of another treatment. Often commenting about the treatments they had received prior feeling like some cold dead pill, non-feeling and heartless merely ushering them in and out of the office like cattle.

They received words of hope and prayer even if in the most meager sense often with open hands and hearts eager almost children-like to see, with what good things these unexpected treatments might bring, the gift went both ways? So I began to apply it in the most rudimentary sense, surrounding the patients with imagery and sounds that spoke of peace, goodness, faith, love, and freedom. The effect on the treatment outcomes was astonishing, instantly beginning to see results and hear reports of people experiencing immediate improvements some even before any physical procedure occurred.

You begin to find a greater and more concentrated effect when words were associated with the treatment application. Thus when a person would express in words the goodness that is attempted to be displayed in touch, one is given the expected outcome in a sort of positive reinforcement, the effect is almost always strengthened, consistent, and seems to be more long-lasting.

But what about when the damage had already been done?

"So ok, now here we sit, the bug bites you on the leg and leaves, what now?"

Healing like wisdom rains down all of the children constantly and continually like the random droplet falling on the parched dry ground of a summers desert day, we people decide two things; first whether or not to actually take the gift as it rains down and then what exactly to do with it.

The first thing we need to do is ensure we don't keep getting bitten over and over again. One must make sure we don't continue to revisit the place that caused us the injury in the first place.

We all walk through gardens of life, stepping stones that waver along a path of our own choosing. Often stepping off the path even for a moment to enjoy the creation along the way whether be it laying in the grass, or partaking of a flower that we happen to glance at as we walk. These actions of creations all have effects on the universe around us because in essence we can create events forever realized, as ripples through still waters, these subconscious yet physical vents have real effects good and bad on the surrounding universe we constantly re-create.

How often have I seen in the course of my career people leaving the office with the necessary information they need to overcome, sometimes even with a complete alleviation of symptoms relating to the injury altogether, just to return a day or two later with the exact returning injury, or to return only a few months later with a similar injury in another spot? In many cases knowing exactly what situation precipitated the issue in the first place, yet these same people then go right back to action or place in their life where the issue occurred in the first place, just to have the same symptoms happen again.

This seems to happen because people first don't see the injury as a product of their occurrence in time, or a test to produce a new and renewed victory, merely a result of bad luck. It is this mentality that has had an effect on the whole, basically taking the miraculous out of healing and perpetuating an increasing ideology of fear, maybe this is the true purpose?

People seem to have this return to the bowl mentality that causes the issue in the first place. I guess changing lifestyles is among the most difficult things anyone can do.

It is basically the purpose of the model of today's Western medicine to perpetuate fear, and it's this stepping away from Faith that actually not only leads to attracting more attacks but leads to voluntary enslavement of our lives as its atmosphere or posture.

The worst is that this fear perpetuates a realization of the very thing people fear, especially when they continually voice, or speak this thing into reality with their own lives, with their very own words. Words can create reality.

I have recently heard it said that this kind of thinking sounds like the power of positive attraction, positive reinforcement, or positive thinking? But if the positive attraction is the repetitive speaking of positive things into one's life, when and if we apply these same teachings to health one would think the same thing applies. God did create all good things, even every positive word. Positive words have been proven to change the very molecular composition of water, so how can we not believe it would have an effect on our bodies, our very health, and wellness, which by the way is made up in the majority by water?

Those like so many gifts God has rained down on all His

children are only a piece of the creation, and if you want to understand and apply them to the whole then you must examine the whole and consider it complete. If you receive a gift from God such as healing, peace, love, or faith then you must recognize where it comes from otherwise the gift can become veiled in the pride and desires of the earth. Applying sound, or water, or light, or touch, healthy natural foods, or positive active directions of movement, if these are all the same then why not apply techniques to bring them all in simultaneously and guarantee all aspects of invasion recovered allowing no darkness in?

In essence, it where you store your treasures you receive? "You can store them on earth where there is rust, worms, and thieves, or you can store them in heaven where there is no rust, no worm to eat, no thief to steal."

I was told of a man who received a six-month prognosis even with chemo and radiation and then only given a fifty percent chance to live the six months. He said to the doctor if I am going to die anyway why not go out doing what I have always wanted instead of living in misery for the last six months with chemo. So he sold everything, quit his overstressed job, packed up his wife and himself, and moved to Grease where he always wanted to retire and live out his days maybe in a vineyard, drinking wine, eating cheese, and living.

If I have to choose how to live my last six months," he told them, "then I choose to live them and not die with them!"

The doctor said if you do that you won't make it six months. That was now over twenty years ago, and he is still going strong, feeling better than ever, drinking wine, and loving life. All the doctors who predicted he wouldn't make it six months are already dead, and he lives, really live!

The positive words have such an influence on the outcomes of the treatments especially the effects. Many people will come in and ask; "can you help take away my pain?" Not realizing that in the same sentence in which they ask for the issue to be removed, they also claim it as their own! Why would you want to remove the system that is warning you about an issue, remove the issue!

"I Am is the greatest single power in the universe, for it is a manifested confession of God Himself."

If we really are created in the image of God, and our very words have creative potential, especially in our own lives, then the act of stating "I Am" this or that would and could be a very potentially realizing action that may have greater consequences on us than we could fathom merely with our physical senses? At what point does a man who tells himself he is a winner or a loser for that matter becomes one, first in his own mind, and then perpetuated throughout the world that directly surrounds him.

Apply this to health care, and the statement to people moving forward is; never even let the words come out of your mouth except for that which you would see yourself become. Nothing negative, belittling, minimizing, or labeling, and especially nothing that states you are anything short of what you were created to be; healthy, happy, loved, and created in the image of God Himself.

When you claim to be someone such as this kind of patient or that, giving yourself, or even accepting labels others place upon you, it is at this moment you basically become what you command. So stop, and you might go one step further, tell others they can keep their curses to themselves, for you refuse to accept them!

Noticing over the course of a career in healthcare a sort of shift in how things were realized especially in the media, among colleagues, or it may have even been how things were subtly taught in schools, a slow yet steady progression of ideology whereby people began to accept the negative proclamations of sicknesses and basically take them upon themselves as simple as accepting a number on their forehead or on the wrist. Earlier I can remember stating that people were afflicted with this or that, and even came down with a particular injury or sickness, now people for the most state they "have" something or they are this or that, referring to themselves with the name of particular sicknesses they feel they have gotten.

This shifting in belief is a dark and diabolical lie designed to enslave God's people in their afflictions and present them powerless and in chains to the malevolent dark spirits that wish to destroy their souls.

That is especially true in the last ten years or so in the health care area, I noticed when people began to believe they have become something, while they may wish for their symptoms to be alleviated, they had not the slightest fraction of hope to think they could be cured. They were already told by doctors there was no cure, the sickness was permanent, terminal, there was nothing that could be done about it, whether it was the doctor telling them, the TV, or even something they read on the internet, they believed it.

Calling yourself a diabetic instead of saying; I am suffering from diabetes is the same as giving up on fighting and just taking it without a fight. What about all the other labels?

"You are what you claim you are. Anything less than a child of God is an insult."

Labels have become the mainstay and as I look back it was almost as subtle as a snake the way it progressed through the medical society and field of medicine as a whole. As I mentioned earlier, there was the formulation of diagnosis codes, whereby a number would be placed on a person identifying them with a particular sickness that people through symptom identification would be suffering from. The very person in order to receive a healthcare benefit had to accept the code as a table with their issue, and with this table came a corresponding name.

No care, prescription, healthcare benefit, or authorization would be granted without the corresponding diagnosis code being placed upon a patient. Then once the code was given the corresponding treatment could not be deviated from regardless of the personal aspects or symptoms a particular person might demonstrate. Patients, in essence, became what they were labeled.

People became amputees instead of suffering from an injury that resulted in an amputation. They became migraine patients instead of suffering from a migraine. Every sort of label of people was created as people became total knee patients, total hips, stroke patients, cancer patients, all of the issues that seemed earlier merely to be products of something else.

People stopped believing they were suffering from addictions and started believing they were addicts, obese, had high blood pressure, are depressed rather than suffering from depression, that they are disabled!

There are no more patients, there are no more terminally ill, only God has the right to determine when a person shall live or die, and only God who creates every day new decides how each of us are to live. We get to decide what we want to look at whether it be the life, light, and everything good in our day, or what we don't have basically the shadows, the negative, the labels placed on us by darkness.

When people stop seeing it as something they are being afflicted with, but something they have become, they, in essence, stop seeing themselves as overcomers, bowing down in submission and just take it. This is what must stop.

"You are not created to be slaves, but to become Kings and Queens."

Words have power, it begins with people letting go of the labels, people need to change their own thinking about themselves even if it merely with words. Some of the first therapeutic procedures one would be having the people do was to merely refer to themselves with good, uplifting, or positive words, and notice I didn't say; "patients," because we need to start telling people not to refer to themselves as patients any longer, but people who are under attack.

"When you speak of the symptoms you happen to be suffering from, do just that speak of them as if the symptoms are something afflicting you from outside of yourselves because they are?" Even though the pain might be inside a person, pain is merely a signal that something else is occurring, it is that precipitating action or event which needs to stop!

"First, turn on the light, then speak the truth."

Returning to the Same Bowl

Very early in my private practice, a lady by the name of Lupe came in who was suffering repeatedly with pain in her low back. Lupe was a sweet person who turned out to be afflicted with a lingering and long-term low back pain stemming from years of progressive degenerative disc disease, eventually causing her to resign her life to filing for disability, stopping work, and using a pain pill or two at least two-three times a week as the pain got too bad for her to hardly function.

We began, as we had been taught and practiced so many times before to work on her by trying to find some specific locations of intermittent tightness and pain. The symptoms would come and go depending on the day, some pain when directly pressing on the exact area of the injury, but not enough to stop her from starting a program of exercise and therapy that could reduce pain, and allow her to build the muscles and structures around the injury to take the pressure off. At this point in my career, we were not yet looking at any possible cause except possibly a direct trauma that may occur with lifting, a fall, or some kind of movement that put pressure on the afflicted tissue, maybe a structural insufficiency such as short muscles, or curvature of the spine, any gambit of other symptoms we would haphazardly try to place blame on for the sudden awakening of symptoms in her.

The program went well, and Lupe often reported the issue completely disappearing by the time she would leave the clinic, just to return the next day or two later. This becomes very perplexing, because while our treatment allowed her the freedom from the pain medication, to an extent when her back pain would return she would come back for treatment and receive relief again now depending on another sort of outside application.

The obvious question was; "what was she doing at home that seemed to re-agitate her back?" At least at that time, enough wisdom was educated to venture this question in the mix? "Nothing out of the normal" she would report, all she was doing was watching her grandchild while her daughter was working, but this was something she had been doing for years and for many others of her children.

"Are you lifting the child, perhaps as the child gets older this is placing a strain on your back?" I then asked.

She assured me she never lifted him but the pain seemed to

return either immediately when she babysat or directly after. Not a day went by when Lupe didn't desperately ask for healing in every way possible, physically, to God with her own mouth, and even believed it was her right to receive it.

While she loved her grandchildren, she often complained about the fact that while she raised her own children, and quite early in her own life, now she seemed to have to raise her grandchildren! It would seem her kids have the babies, then drop them over to her for their care, and she left carrying the burden one after another!

Had I known then what I know now, I would have realized that her issue came not only physically on her back, but also had a spiritual side to the injury; that the pain was an attack on the vulnerable area of her life, her desperate need to carry the burdens of her family to the point where she will even risk her own health? She would heal each time she came in, each time she seemed to receive full relief and a return of full function, just to a return back to the very issue that caused the problem in the first place.

Lupe was not willing to let go of that anger against her children and ultimately herself for allowing herself to get in this pickle in the first place. And while she so desperately desired to be free of the pain, and possible enslavement the pain pills offered to her for her health, economic well-being, and even her own self-image, she kept going back to the bowl that caused her problem in the first place.

This back and forth returning, to and from pain, repeated itself over the course of almost six months until her insurance company finally stopped authorizing her to come in. She often knew and even stated she knew that physically she really wasn't able to take care of her grandchildren as she did, but just couldn't bring herself to the point where she would tell her children. Eventually, Lupe gave up and resigned herself to the life she had, pain, pain pills, and taking care of the babies of her babies.

I think we have come far enough in our analysis to realize that at least a realization of where the window is in her life, would be the first step in closing it off for the purpose of stopping the repeated attacks. In this case, the prescription would be for Lupe to forgive her children and herself for the pickle! The next time the symptoms come knocking on the door of her back, simply tell them to leave! Sit back and see what happens.

Recently I worked on a man by the name of Peter and while he really didn't do anything that may have precipitated an injury to his back suddenly and spontaneously he sustained severe pain in the low back. When he went in for X-rays it turned out he had a compression fracture to the low back and the backbones of the spine were pressing on the nerve causing severe pain in the leg.

After immediately commanding the attacker to leave, at which time he did feel some improvement, also other preparations were conducted that resulted in placing Godly and natural remedies immediately to the injured area. Normally for a compressed disc, the only medical procedure recommended is surgery to remove the pressure from the nerve, resulting in one or more fused discs of the low back. This procedure not only is painful but only seems to actually help maybe slightly over fifty percent of the time due to the fact that the irritation of the nerves was already present.

We also immediately determined when asking God for advice that he had been carrying an extreme increase of burden in his low back mentally as well as spiritually and worried about the decisions he was making regarding the people who placed these burdens on him.

"Lights on, window found."

We asked for God to forgive him and the people placing these burdens on him, asking that God would close the window the attack is coming in. We also went on to pray that the body would flush the damage the injury caused with pure blessed water, and Lion of Judah anointing oil being dubbed on the surface of his back, then clean up the mess that the attack already did?

Within moments he began to feel some immediate improvement, and in a few days, the injury began to subside to the point where he no longer needed pain pills. After only a little over one month, Peter has been re-examined and found that the fracture has completely and miraculously healed, relieving the pressure off the nerve, and other than a little residual stiffness, the problem has completely disappeared. So much so, that Peter recently shoveled his own driveway, quite a feat for a man in his mid-eighties who recently broke his back, or so he had been told?

Peter while he saw what the attack had done to him physically, refused to admit or even hear any mention of a Broken back in reference to himself. He let his faith dictate what he knew and what his body realized, and in response mobilized the God Gene inside of himself to receive full and miraculous healing from God.

While he still had contact with the people who were placing burdens on him, he was cautious not to let them too close until they could reduce their own pressures on him, thus perhaps the reason the aching issues still lingered?

Address the Causes, all the causes are key for effective and total victory against attack!

Once you have accepted the idea that you are not powerless in your quest to fight back against an assault of an illness or injury, and nothing is certain especially the doomsday advice that is given by people who either by miss-guided education or alternative motives for having you feel enslaved or helpless in your life, victory is as easy as lifting up ones head and asking.

Another simple truth about health care is that unless a person looks to the cause of an issue, and then concentrates on a subsequent treatment plan to fight the affliction in a likewise rehabilitation plan, they have a blind man in a boxing matches chance of overcoming the attack or sickness.

If a person doesn't know where the attack is coming from, then how can they possibly know how to fight?

The evidence and manipulation are all around us, constantly coming at us in every possible form, presenting a complete bombardment of attempted poisoning of our bodies through our eyes, ears, mouths, minds, and bodies with one purpose, to manipulate, negatively affect, weaken our body, at the same time confuse and lie to our minds, distracting us from the truth, eventually manipulate our beliefs to the point where we give up all freedom and become slaves to the temple for any health or hope.

Blessed for us as Jesus Himself said; *"It is not what goes into a man's mouth that corrupts humbug what comes out that corrupts."*

Being myself a trained martial artist, it grants a bit of an advantage to, if nothing else, understand the subtle similarities of battling sicknesses spiritually and using trained as well as understood methods shown successfully in the physical, for common knowledge is by definition common. For example; a person doesn't have to be thoroughly trained in the higher disciplines of self-defense to know a person doesn't bring a simple knife to a sword fight, or maybe better illustrated an aspirin to battle with a legion of spirits!

If you want to fight a spiritual being you must use spiritual weapons, such as those given us by God Himself! If you are going to a bug-fight, you have your shoe, most of the time that is enough!

Back to the simple statement about whether or not one might seek the cause? When seeking, or what exactly everyone knows to be the truth about sicknesses is removed from them and placed into the hands of others, in fact, the result is that the control is removed from the person.

First and foremost in the present healthcare system with its basic pharmaceutical-insurance-driven presentation that seems to care nothing about curing anybody of anything, hopelessness is sown like weeds in a beautiful garden? They demonstrate it daily in their ads which clearly address and speak of interest in treating the symptoms of the afflictions we suffer from, making money, and enslaving us into a belief system of total dependency and continual usage. The basic fact is, there is not a single medicine on the market that cures anybody of anything, they all merely reduce the symptoms that the injuries or sicknesses cause, and we sit back, hope, even pray that sickness will then just go away, but in this is the prayer, we are intact praying for the symptoms to go away.

The public is told that millions are being spent on finding

cures, but who is doing the research, seems to be the very companies that profit the most by us using their medicines are the ones doing the research, or at least funding the programs and determining in which direction this research will head? This is especially true for the various ailments that have seemed to rear their ugly heads over the last few years, promises of cures are always just tests, months, on the brink, or just beyond the horizon away, but the deeper we look into healthcare research, the more examples that the majority of research actually is in finding drugs that reduce symptoms, while at the same time, maintain the affliction so it is necessary for the patient to continue taking the drug for as long as possible, and in some case facilitating one or two others that we will then need to take more medicine to counter the new symptoms arising?

Cures and reports of cures are reported by the media to be researched all over the world, and if one happens to be found it is quickly swooped up by the pharmaceutical companies, attempted to synthesize for its useful ingredients, and then ultimately shelved. Many non-addictive sleeping aids, pain remedies, blood pressure, diabetes remedies, even cancer cures have been reported only to disappear suddenly as new breakthroughs seem to linger just on the horizon. I can honestly say that I have treated countless people who have either reported by direct experience or have first-hand knowledge of this or that natural plant, a combination of natural products, or a program that cured them or someone they knew from a seemingly incurable illness, then only later to have the information quietly and diabolically removed from access, from the internet or any other reporting entity, as if it had never existed at all?

Conspiracy? One might think so, even dare to say so?

I have an old friend and since he is one of the most prominent neurosurgeons in the world I will not even venture to give his initials. But let's just say he developed a procedure that saves children's lives from a most dilapidating injury of the neck, large tumors that cause paralysis, and in most cases death.

I had lunch with him quite a while ago, and he spoke of an odd factual report of when he first developed this procedure, the cases of these tumors were so rare that he would fly all over the world to treat maybe a couple cases a year, with amazing success I might add. Over the course of the decades to follow the cases became more and more frequent, to the point where he would schedule one a week every week for the last couple of years and never had to leave the United States. As a matter of fact, there are so many of these cases today he needed to train others how to perform this delicate procedure just to address the many that have sprung up?

Conspiracy, what we are feeding our children? What we are attracting with our fear? A growing spirit? All I know is even as we sat to speak of such possibilities, I could see in his face, his own fear to even speak of this possible spiritual element, for fear he might be excommunicated for merely suggesting such a thing?

Our basic beliefs are constantly being challenged.

In a time not so long ago if a person started suffering from an illness they did just that, they "came down" with, suffered from, or caught this or that? Now people are told they "Are Sick" instead of suffering from a sickness. This is a very slight and mild form of manipulation of the mind, significant because if a person now believes they "Are" or have become something within themselves, instead of merely "suffering" from something, they tend to give up hope, and relinquish much easier their own willingness to fight, the result; they will just sit there and take it as the abusive suffering, or worse yet returning attacks' continue.

Yet as a medical practitioner I too have been an active participant in this sense of the brainwashed helplessness that we are being dowsed unto these people continually when all they are looking for is a little help with their infirmities. It was my own participation and even the guilt of having profited from this sustained dogma of misguided information that I will have to live with for the rest of my life.

"I would at his point publicly confess to you and ask anyone who may have been misled by my own past healthcare suggestions to forgive me, as I ask God to forgive myself for my participation in this part. And finally, I will forgive myself for being led down a path that I knew at the time seemed suspiciously tainted in greed and pride."

This most recent helpless social manifestation is truly a new occurrence pressing to the forefront over the last ten or fewer years. I remember only just a few years ago, people would come to me with a preconceived notion that they were suffering from this or that issue, no matter if it was a direct orthopedic dramatic event such as a break or injury, or if they were suffering from a more complex systemic affliction such pain in the back, a new total knee replacement surgery performed on them, a recent heart attack, a pending or recent amputation, or an attack of any "name" such as Lupus or High Blood Pressure, and could almost exactly pinpoint in most cases the exact day the issue started, thus leading to a possible examination as to the cause, at least at the time in the most basic sense, with its own possible cure wishes and hopes, this seemed at least then to be the standard procedure?

Now, today, people come and say; "I have this or that", "I have a Rotator Cuff", "I have pain", "I am a cancer patient", "A Diabetic", "Disabled", "An Amputee", "A Schizophrenic", "I AM SICK" having resolved themselves to the belief that these sicknesses are a part of who they are, who they have become and finally who they were created to be! They have given up all hope to a possible cure, mostly because they have been told they are incurable, and merely seek treatment to help them function with this new life's sentence.

Amazingly; People who believe they are sick usually are, or on their way to becoming so, and either first experience even the slightest warning symptom such as a sneeze or a fear that some Boogy-Man is hiding in a cookie, then immediately start speaking it, immediately begin believing it, and suddenly it is realized in their soul. Yet those who refuse to believe they are sick, speak the contrary ultimately prove not to be.

This fact would lend to the statement that the mind has a much greater effect on the body than the body on the mind itself, and the spirit, which you believe has the greatest almost infinite influence on both.

If an attack is merely an image we place on ourselves, then the weapon is a new image spoken in words of faith, health, freedom, and most importantly Godliness.

If the attacks come in the form of visions, dark shadows, or giants who only look big because they are being projected on the walls of our should house, then put positive images of health before your eyes only! Flood your eyes with God-given natural beauty, smiles, healthy, pure, and noble words that penetrate your eyes envisions of Godly promises of life and love.

If an affliction or storm is caused by negative or destructive actions, place positive and uplifting actions in the place of your path, choose another path, no matter how risky or scary change may seem? Any direction away from the dark and toward light is good and can only be met with an increase in your soul?

Good natural foods, clean healthy water, clean fresh air, truths, positive words, uplifting stories, a child's love, the devotion of a pet, all are freely given by God for us merely to use.

If you want to receive complimentary attributes of which you totally deserve, give them to others, give them to yourself "For God's Sake."

If you want help, help others, if you want peace then grant it to others, if you want Good and healthy food to be used by your body, give to others. *"Give and ye shall receive"*

If you want a better workplace then make it better yourself one step at a time with one small action, one single positive word makes it better than it was before. Give that which you would have for yourself to others and it is in effect given to God, of which no man can God be in debt to. Once you know why, or in what way you are attacked, fighting becomes clear and easy.

And if you want to be assured of constant and sustainable victory then do them all!

Speak It Into Reality

So the first exercise or thing that must happen in the therapeutic process of injury recovery is a vocal manifestation of what we are expecting. Believe it has become manifest even in word, act upon it, and then witness the increase in our life in response. Any progress is progress! Basically, command the attack to leave.

People have trouble understanding that each and every moment of life is a gift, and as such, there is truly something perfect and godly to experience even in a single breath, but it is the worries and troubles of the world, its responsibilities, and pondering, that has robbed people of the gifts they could experience if they just stopped and saw them.

I myself have been so guilty of these worries and anxieties whether they be with pain, financial problems, storms, tragedies, whatever, they always have the effect of taking my eyes off the world around me and placing them on the very small, and often yet to materialized worry, that of which I happen to be dwelling on at that moment. Worry is nothing else but the fixation on what is not, the staring at the shadow trying to decide if there is substance to it or not, and the contemplation of every factor that might lead to the shadow actually taking form? That would seem the very thing a shadow or dark spirit would want if especially if it feeds or gains its substance from this feared devotion?

The solution is an active and conscious decision not to look at negative, shadows, or worry but look up and out into the world around to see the light of the gift God has given right at this moment. Maybe even command yourself not to worry? But better yet, why even use the word? Speaking the word in the sentence, "I don't want to worry" in essence creates in you the thing you speak; granted you receive the ability "not to want" something and that something, in this case, is "worry."

A better approach is to thank God for the solution of the problem you are looking for even before it arrives; such as "Thank you God for that perfect job you brought me, and all the abundance that it has given my family." "Thank you for scaring away the darkness that is knocking at my throat or nose, thank you for the light and the promise that the light does scare away the darkness, that you for the victory and the infinite gifts You give in every breath of this life."

Yes, that sounds much better.

Did He not say; *"Go your faith has made you whole"?*

When it comes to people suffering from injury the instruction becomes one of reinforced positive experience on every point of experience possible, basically sight, sound, taste, and smell, even feeling. Feel the soft touch of the loving partners' caress and realize the pain has gone. Inject good into any situation and it becomes better! If a problem causes you to experience something or magnifies it, then the solution is doing the opposite you are feeling it is driving you to?

For example; the attack of depression has an effect on the majority of individuals to cause them to de-socialize or withdrawal from contacting other individuals, and likewise, if you want to really effectively treat depression on a therapeutic level then re-socialization is paramount for helping these people obtain final and long-lasting victory. Give and it will be given unto you.

So by vocalizing the healing, that we have been promised the victory is received, the actual creation in our spoken voice puts into place the positive motion of the reality created.

So often as it is seen in the common medical community,

people have become fearful of the unseen and cruel sicknesses that seem to lurk in the shadows of their lives. These pour souls then contract a simple symptom such as a bite, a harsh touch, or inkling of rebellion in their body, at which time their minds immediately go to the worst-case scenario, looking even believing they have contracted the worse sicknesses? They speak negativity into themselves, and with their words, their every thought, in a state of fear go rushing to the doctors who are quick to label it, label them, search for it, or test for it. People pray to God "It" hasn't already become what they already are claiming with their many words, thoughts, and fears to be.

These poor victims may feel a twinge in their chest or pain in their head, somewhere along the way they left a door open to their inner-house or stepped into a hole and a little creature bit them.

Doubt turns into fear, fear into self-cursing, ultimately they draw the curse, the dark shadow, the storm to themselves like a wild animal is drawn to a fearful rabbit trembling under a tree, or worse yet, they speak it unto others who are around them, under their responsibility, such as with children or loved ones and unknowingly project that fear unto them, making them then targets. Fear is the catnip of the spiritual world.

These poor fearful souls go to people who they trust to tell them the answers, people who have been given authority to find and know the answers. Unfortunately, these very people they go to are unfortunately the same ones taught by the industries, philosophies, or spirits, basically that they want all of us to put our trust not in God, in oil-based drugs or practices of darkness that enslave us and wish to rob us of every good thing our Father God has freely given us. These same practices only seem to enslave us, fill us with doubt, or lead us onto a road of depression, poverty, and ultimately death.

One after another these poor individuals are given drugs and instructed, or pressed upon, or in some cases as in the innocents forced upon them, to put every foul sort of toxin of the world in their mouths in a feeble attempt to try to elevate some initial symptom. These very symptoms are merely the warning sign that our own body is attempting to fight off the would-be attack! This symptom, this sneeze, stuffy nose, headache, or chill, being nothing more than an alarm bell to warn us of an issue or cause, so unaffected by the drug we are taking, that these same causes maybe even in some cases can be precipitated or even enhanced by the same said usage, overuse, or dependency on the drug? Many of the drugs we take while they may reduce the symptoms that arise from the attacks, actually weaken our bodies, and thus allow for what would appear to be a greater opening of the very doors that the attacking creatures are coming into our souls home through.

"God gives us everything we need to overcome every obstacle this life might seem to place in our way."

What does this mean? We are given in this life each and every day we open our eyes all the things we need to overcome the challenges of that day? Perhaps it means we have already been given everything in this life we may need to overcome any physical infirmity at hand, we merely have to reach out and use it.

"Both! That is exactly what it means!"

People think that life, especially the body is everything, then the mind controls the body actions and events, a little less, and finally, the spirit is the least significant part floating somewhere apart or on your shoulder whispering softly in your ear. That being said, it is also believed that medicines that have a dramatic effect on the body must be the solution for all the issues of the body?

Yes, that would be true if we were merely flesh and bone, but we are more than flesh, we are more than minds, and as we have already seen we are primarily and for the most infinite part spirits. Spirits while being slightly influenced by earthly poisons, are only on the most fractional basis influenced by the physical poisons of a single day. This concept is no different than dropping a single drop of poison into the sea, what effect does it really have on the whole ocean?

"Only a Spirit can attack a spirit!"

These dark spirits hate God's children so, not the germs, not the foolish vessels that we think are doing this to us, do we really think that germs actually have a notion we even exist? They have no more awareness of us than a carpet-mite is aware of the skyscraper the carpet happens to lie in? Germs don't hate us, as a matter of fact, we coexist with many needing the very nutrients they produce in our intestines to build strong resistances to storms of all kinds. No, it's the dark spirits that drive them to their own destructive purposes that hate us, and thus it is these ruling agents hiding yet directing from the seemingly distant trees, these are the creatures that need to have our attention and counter-attacks.

The fear of the attack, or the memories of attacks of the past, have the most long-lasting effects on our own lives. Not the foolish scorpions being used to their own destruction, stinging once, then waiting almost foolishly patient as they themselves seem in a loss of recognition that we will dish out infinitely greater destructive forces than their little bodies could possibly take? No, the spirits that drive them, these are the real enemies.

In the Roman army days, the leaders, the ones actually driving the armies, telling them who to attack, where exactly they must direct their efforts, and even the very moment and in what fashion the attack must occur, these so-called decision-makers would cowl in the trees, hiding in the bushes just beyond the battlefield close enough to see the action yet far enough away to first not be seen, and second, have an avenue to make a quick retreat of escape if things didn't seem to progress well. As much as self-spoken or written stories, would speak of generals fighting alongside their troops in the front lines, these are but stories and the actual leaders of legions were nothing more than sniveling cowards, many would not even carry sharpened swords as to not risk cutting themselves? Basically, they were harmless physically only being powerful in their threats and ability to elicit fear.

In the natural, it always represents the supernatural, and if this is the case then the attacking agent is not in the germ, or in the bat that is about to hit said head, but lingering somewhere close enough to be seen yet far enough away to run if detected? This is important information when said light turns on and you look for a possible cause to the attack, then why now information?

What exactly is going on, who is watching, what are you busy with, thinking, doing at the very moment you feel a symptom your body is reacting to? The moment of awareness? And if you can not identify anything specific then ask God to show you, and thus react no matter what it is.

Back to healing, in life, as in health and wellness, people have basically two choices; they can be persons dancing through the beautiful garden of life looking at every beautiful flower in their garden as they head towards the light, or they can sit in the dirt staring at their little toe wondering in oblivion why it hurts even though they just watched the scorpion run away or cower in the corner like the coward it is.

"When you are a person who looks to God for life, and every stone in which to step as you pass through your own garden which is your soul, that which is a beautiful one, a special one, that you absolutely know was created only for you, then you have absolutely nothing to fear because God the

Great I Am is with you."

Did He not say; *"My rod and staff will comfort you?"*

So if we see or know of a bully lurking down a particular street, or hiding in a bush, and choose to take another path, we must at the very least, not fear. I have noticed through my own experiences that on occasion I might find myself on the wrong path or direction in life and suddenly I am at times granted a brief but somewhat fearful warning like the hair-raising in the back of my head, time to move or go someplace else?

"This, I have found, is God's messenger or an angel gently warning me of impending dangers or attacks. For those who are trying to listen to God, not being completely distracted by complications or the misguided necessities of the world around them, these gentle nudges or signs come daily as people quickly run through the fields of God's glorious creation for them each and every moment of a day."

Here again, look up, and speak into your life the reality of what you want. Let's get back to the best way, people should deal with sicknesses? Once stung, what should a person do about it, if they know they happen to have been bitten?

We have already realized that lifting up the head and after turning on the light, there is a promised realization of the truth, this seeking the wisdom, asking for help, represents an active and positive choice to seek Light in a persons life and facilitates them immediately upon the road to healing. Then what next?

It is said we must *"put on the full armor of God."* So *this* next action would represent an active choice to do something physical such as picking up the tools to defend yourself. God provides the rod and staff, you can call to angels for help, this can never hurt, turning on the bright light is basically a great battle plan, creatures of the night always run away from bright light. God has given us tools merely through His written Word, but also by way of promise, grants to us the means to find what we need to overcome, even within ourselves, basically the initiation of the God Gene.

The world has made people afraid of light, with all the UV scare and everything else, getting people to cover up completely, only go out at night, hide in the dark, sunblock this, sunshade that, stick their head in the sand, most of the time looking to something good, natural, or simply seems to be the opposite of what is instructed to us our whole life especially in the medical community? I have even over the last couple of years seen more and more examples of people being prescribed chemotherapies, exploratory surgeries, correctional procedures, or other extremely dangerous, and expensive I may add, treatment methods when no detected affliction or other harmful issues has yet been detected, and in some cases merely as a preventative measure just in case a person might acquire it someday? This is the definition of creating fear!

Light is never a bad thing, Light is from God and it is good, and while everything that is used in excess can be an issue in our lives, to be told when you have an affliction you must actually place yourself into darkness as a way to remedy it, seems to me to be the equivalent of asking a devil to chase out a devil?

Now Water is the best and most abundant physical component for healing, and any therapeutic process or mopping up session should use water as a key ingredient in this process. Be a fireman, turn on the water and direct it, a good water hose can scare any animal away much more effectively than any gun, but only if there is water coming out of the hose.

"Water is a good start."

Touch My People

When given the question, and wondering about a possibility of healing someone, almost from the first moment of awareness people associate the thought of healing with the sense of touch, being that which people need to initiate in order to facilitate the healing process.

If we consider the natural world and look carefully, it is almost immediately clear with each and every injury a person responds almost naturally and immediately to touch.

A Mothers' child hurts themselves, and the mother almost instinctively takes the child and kisses the hurt, caresses them, or holds them in a comforting manner, embellishing love, giving compassion, and fulfilling comfort. The child receives this and immediately responds, there is an immediate calming of irritation, a relaxing of tension, and a realization that everything will be all right. I myself as a father have had almost an undeniable need to embellish my own children with love especially when they are hurt, what is amazing is the reciprocation of love that I immediately feel when I give or get this back from them. And if I, or a mother for that matter, can give with my own limited love how much more would The Father in Heaven, who loves with infinitely more give His children who come to Him when they are hurt?

Science would say the stimulation of fine touch nerves overwhelms the slower pain receiving nerves and the pain is not felt as the child receives a comforting stimulus instead of pain? But I would like to also believe the child receives love in the way of warmth transmitted in real perceivable energy by the mother in the form of caring emotional love being given through her concern, love, and compassion. The waters of the body pass this information through the entirety of the soul as a drop is dispersed throughout the invite reaches of an ocean immediately.

This feeling of warm communicated love the child feels this deep within them no different than the mother does in return and experiences it not merely as only a superficial warming sensation on the skin but as a totally penetrating radiating a feeling of love that perpetually courses through to the bone, to the very foundations of a person's soul. A belief is expressed and generated in the form of love, life, peace, and joy, and all these feeling overpower the recent feelings of destruction, pain, fear, and sadness. Light blazes and shadows flee!

"Inject love and the darkness must immediately flee."

I decide to put this to the test and began to see if the people could actually feel when I was truly was expressing a feeling of concern, and wondered if they were aware of such feelings at all, especially if unexpressed by me. The only thing I could think of was asking within myself was a simple prayer as I laid my hands on them.

As I earlier said while I was not in my opinion one who considered himself a praying individual, a simple; "Please help this person" seemed all I needed, and the concentration of wanting the person to feel the warmth with this statement as I laid my hand on them even for the most simple massaging technique, seemed to be sufficient to elicit an immediate and palatable warmth response from the person being treated.

I was amazed at the reactions of the people, they almost always immediately became aware that my hands became warmer and even in many cases hot, feeling a sort of deep heating experience much deeper and more pronounced than they had ever felt before, especially aware of this sensation since I had started treating them?

But what now, did the people when they felt this warmth, did they heal? Many often felt better, some significantly better, even to the point to where the pain or irritation would simply disappear, but often and in many cases the pain would only reappear later or the next day and the person would come back for another of the same experience of relief. This left me with only more questions, what is the purpose of this revelation, and how could it be used in the process of helping heal people?

"Warmth you felt in your hands and so many others who have had a calling into the healing arena is a gift, a sign that they are engaging in a path of righteousness. Everyone who has been healed is called then in their own turn to help heal others, this is how the healing gene is engaged and mobilized."

I have over the course of my years heard of and even met many who have received this gift of "healing hands," some have even been hailed as healers, but in many the gift was not sustainable, working for some and not for others, this too is a perplexing issue to consider, especially when these same people later come to light as being perpetrators of hoaxes or frauds merely as a means to extort sums of money from believing and gullible crowds.

"God's blessing rain down on all His children's heads like raindrops being scattered in the winds, regardless of the boundaries, whether they be countries, races, or even religions. Men place these boundaries on each other attributing some qualifiers as if God's love needs a qualifier. If God has given life to any and all of the children of the world, would He not rain down blessing also indiscriminately?"

It is when these individuals have received one or more blessings, such as the honor of being used by God to heal another individual, and then take this honor upon themselves somehow believing that the healing powers come from them instead of God, it at the moment I believe they have elevated themselves above God and then God either removes the ability for them to command the action, or they try to command in their own name and not God's, resulting in nothing happening.

The foolish practitioners of their own reported healing attributes, either become blinded by the veils of the world or remain blind in their own journeys far off the paths of light and the life God would create for them.

Unfortunately for many of these healers, they seem to fall the victim to vanity, finding the need to regurgitate the healing event for a paying audience. This is a slander against God, and the spirits that drive vanity, greed, and lust for power, have one goal of their own existence, and that is to be seen, lure followers away from God and destroy the gifts of God.

Yet I have also experienced practitioners of true or God-centered faith when receiving the healing gift, whether being healed themselves or students of healing instructions, experience a true desire to be a part of this experience at least in their own desire to support the experience in others, or begin to practice it themselves? There seems to be an overwhelming desire to share what they have received, and I believe necessary for bringing the healing process full circle.

Healing is like unto sowing of the seed, and when this then comes on to harvest will grow, multiply and become bountiful even unto feeding many others. Placing it in a jar and burying it in the garden will never allow it to grow.

"The evidence of this is a continuation of their own examination of creation, people who seek light, goodness, and healing for others, seek all of these things for themselves."

Light draws the light, and for all who seek truth, goodness, love, peace, if they look far enough and remove the veils from their eyes of man-made prodigiousness, they will find God calling them.

"That is why one must always remember where true healing comes from, and give credit, where credit is due."

You have heard a simple explanation of what sickness is, healing is just as simple.

Peter Colla

The First Physical Therapist

Physical Therapy in its most basic form is the application of Physical therapeutic applications as a means to rehabilitate or facilitate the healing process in individuals after they have suffered from an injury, whether it be a traumatic event, a post-acute sickness process, or a systemic deviation from the norms of function following one or more breakdown of normal bodily functions, all related to physicality or function.

Practicing Physical Therapy or at least applying the therapeutic techniques to thousands of patients over the course of tens of years, has allowed me to see the relative significance the application of natural stimulus has on the body both in the immediate and long-term basis regarding the return to normal or even possible enhancement of function. It has also allowed me to witness firsthand where the application of physical stimulus by themselves and singularly also results in reduced effectiveness of the applications over a large group of people, thus suggesting for other factors must be involved for a consistent and guaranteed healing outcome, one that far exceeds the mere prescribed and commonly authorized as well as practiced procedures.

As I read and studied more the historical accounts of Jesus Christ it occurred to me, increasingly as I looked at them through the eyes of a medical practitioner, that many of the applications of healing had similarities to many of the applications practiced perhaps inadvertently, at least in part, by the majority of the therapeutic practitioners I had witnessed in the field.

Jesus was the first true healer, healing all parts of the person, not merely the body, but the mind, and the spirit simultaneously.

He seemed to be able to discern with Godly intuition exactly the direction in which to apply the necessary stimulus for the more apparent and qualitative results. He knew exactly what direction and in which realm to operate to get the job done.

It would seem that this is because He understood people are more than just bodies and symptoms, but also the experiences of their minds, and most importantly their spirits, and in considering this, applied the healing to all of these areas proportionally according to the individuals need, healing them not only in their immediate physical areas but completely as to help them on the course to fulfill their own destinies, their very souls?

I have noticed, or better yet have been taught by God, that in every case, some kind of action was coupled with the healing, whether it be "Pick up your mat and walk," "Go report to the teachers of the temple," "Dip yourselves in the Jordan" or merely "Go and sin no more," the bottom line there was always an action coupled with healing. They not only heard His words (physical reality in action), but saw with their eyes the pure Light, witnessed a truly God creation, experiences in many cases physical touch if merely the waves of sound bouncing off their bodies, in some cases got to eat some Godly produced food, drank water turned to wine, made wondrous, and in every case a combination of all of these infused in belief or re-education of the people's believable experience.

"The action places reality into the healing process, not only does the person experience even at the moment a small fraction of improvement, they experience it in their senses; hearing, seeing, tasting, and feeling it is through this positive experience that they that then receive as a physical almost therapeutic momentous experience of healing. There is an exact event created, they have been told, and it is now and forever coupled with their own healing experience, they

thus believe."

Belief is the basis for all reality in the world. I Am is the most powerful force in the entire physical universe, spiritual, mental, or physical. I Am transcends time and space, for what you believe you are you become.

"If a person only believes even with the most insignificant fraction like a mustard seed, then everything is possible, even the impossible."

These are not new revelations, everything you need to understand about healing Jesus has already demonstrated, had documented by his followers, and revealed from the very first moment God physically stepped onto the world stage two thousand years ago.

Exercise has the same effect, and that is why it is such a perfect therapeutic tool for rehabilitation of the boy who suffers and needs to pick up his mat and walk. People often misunderstand exercise seeing it as a sort of program one needs to fulfill to accomplish a specific task. But as a therapist I realize that exercise does not cause the body to grow or heal, the body merely reacts to the stimulus that is being given it, that's why it works with some people, and with others, it doesn't.

If a person wants to walk they merely have to start first believing they are meant to walk, then begin along a path of belief and actions that promotes them to the course of experience which includes walking. Jesus used many examples of exercise, adding movement into the healing process; "pick up your mat and walk," "go down to the Jordan," "go back home your event is already healed," go, go, and again go. Walk down the path, take the first step, head towards someplace, a life-giving place, a healing place.

Perhaps this may have been because the actual moment of healing took place at the instant Jesus showed up, the rest was the after effect the mopping up of the mess. The persons who picked up their mat had to be healed in their minds, or in the very least in their belief, to actually pick up the mat, they believed what they heard, they felt the results of those words on themselves even if it was but a small fraction, a small mustard seed size portion of faith, and acting with the body was only a simple result.

Belief starts a sort of domino effect of sound, using spoken words, resonating around, in between the very particles of our entire existence, in us through us and completely around us, a miraculous change in their very atoms, genes, our very cells, and thus this spontaneous miracle occurs within the bodies anatomical essence-essential moment in time itself.

Sounds like quantum physics, the studying of the most basic particles of the known universe, their movements, interactions, and in some cases their possible origins, and how healing might fit in here?

If Quantum physics is the study of the particles themselves, the healing takes place within the vast space within them, around them, and between them, then healing is merely an expression of physicality on the most basic level, an expression of God Himself. The expression of I Am, the realization of what we are, and the moment of healing instead of admitted defeat, are all the same!

If you snap a dry twig at what moment does the twig break? The moment you hear the snap or the moment you feel it?

It would be said by learning and experience the moment you feel the snap, experience the release of energy, the motion, or hear the sound, simultaneously?

Yet, even in the most sensitive and observant fraction of time it still takes a split second for you to become aware of something after it already occurred, thus the moment is over and forever in the past, leaving you with the feeling of the effect of the action of snapping and the two pieces resting in each hand. So is it with sicknesses, by the time you feel it, it has already happened, dwelling in the past, nothing to fear, your reaction is key for how you are to experience it!

Sicknesses and injuries are exactly the same, and as well so is healing, they all occur in a moment in time transcending the very essence of time and space. What starts out as simple events become reality depending on our awareness.

You only become sick after being in an attack, and then only if you take it upon yourself and believe it to be so. If you make yourself sick with your words, and belief.

God's children are not now, ever were, or ever will be created sick, they can only claim this upon themselves, or have it placed upon them in and this basically represents in the form a sort of curse.

What doesn't kill you makes you stronger?

Peter Colla

Overcoming

If we suppose that everything in this creation is at hand for us to use for the overcoming of any issue people face then you must believe; "Everything You Need" means everything, and every issue not only means the hole, the wolf, the disease, cancer, whatever, but also the effects of the fall!

"God creates all of His children, every single day, with everything they need to overcome every issue they will need throughout that particular day of their life. As a matter of fact, God creates them with everything they need in every single breath!"

The statement "Life in every breath" is commonly taught in various forms of eastern philosophy and martial arts training, but isn't only a Buddhist thought having to do with the search for balance, "War and Peace," training within the fighting skills and balancing them with painting, dance, or poetry, various art practices to create harmony? The search for balance as well as harmony is merely an aspect of the realization of the pureness of natural beauty that resides within each and every observation one may take time to observe in God's entire creation.

"God rains His wisdom as well as his blessings down on all His children heads indiscreetly as a way to show them all His creation, and when they ask the meaning of it. Nothing God shares with any of us is any more or different, than anything He has shared with everyone else, since the beginning of time and likewise over the whole world, the only difference is whether or not you chose to listen, write it down and share it with others."

Many elder patients often mention family traits or things that they did in the past that basically pre-destine them into suffering from issues, but I have seen when people apply the principles as spoken of earlier than use all-natural and God-given elements to facilitate the clean up of the mess almost miraculous healing and even a sort of turning back of the clock restoration occurs.

People will

People are deceived into thinking they are doomed because of the mistakes or abuses of the past, the same way they are also deceived by the misconception that there is nothing they can do about their issue themselves but must look to a more learned and regulated industry to secure any kind of assurance or insurance of health. This goes in direct contradiction to the promise that Christ made us during his time on earth and documented by His examples.

"Overcoming amounts to nothing more than simply stepping up onto the water and walking above the waves in a storm."

For the first time in History people were healed, blind people regained their sight, the dead rose, people of all sorts of afflictions were suddenly or systematically healed. These were documented events that nobody disputes, many of such cases find themselves common occurrences today, I have even personally spoken to many people who have sprung back to life some as a result of medical interventions, others in a few cases even came back with no medical intervention at all, merely because they were told to on the other side.

But nowhere have I ever heard of anyone walking on water.

"When you take control of a storm in your belief, understanding the image, waves, and winds have no effect on you unless you let them, in essence, you step up above the waves and walk on the water."

"All storms no matter what you call them, sickness, disease, addiction, depression, having things stolen from you, losing

a job, all forms of attacks are all the same, merely movements of energies surrounding you and being directed to attack you. Now that you know how insignificant the spiritual energies that direct them are compared to you and the powers God has granted you, stepping out above them is as simple as lifting your head."

Stepping over the attacks is one thing, then choosing what tools will need to be used for the cleaning up or restorations caused by the damage already perpetrated by the storm is another. People still suffer from the aftermath of the bug bite, no matter how small. I knew a man I loved, a dear friend, a good man, who lost a leg because of a bug bite, but it wasn't the bite that suddenly caused the leg to fall off, but the misguided ideology that allowed him to disregard the window he had open in his life, letting in the creature or in this case allowing the spirit to come in and direct the bug to bite him. The bug brought the infection, his disregard to an earlier issue in his life allowed him to minimalist the issue until it caused so much destruction his life was in jeopardy. Even after the leg was gone his inability to address the issues that caused all these problems in the first place finally got the best of him and the journey down the path of this life at least came to an end.

"When the attack occurs and leaves a child with a mess to

clean up, use anything and everything God gives you right at hand to continue to overcome and move further through your garden. As a matter of fact, if the solution to the problem is not at hand, then a person merely has to ask God to reveal it. God will never be shown lie since He promised you will have all you need to overcome if you are meant to overcome then you will?"

I began to instruct the people who came to me to only use natural products as much as they can. Use water in every aspect of the therapeutic process, whether it be baths, pools, wet compresses, or simple flushing with water. Fasting, three-day fasts, or intermittent, all of these were often instructed as well but always in cooperation with using water or baths in conjunction with these. When water could not be confirmed to be clean, do the best a person could to filter it, and when in doubt bless it.

"Water is God's conduit to relay emotions such as love, faith, and belief, Jesus said He was the living waters, and if you bless these waters with your own love they will manifest love whenever, where ever, and in whatever fashion you use them."

Using all forms of goodness in every portal in our being assures us that light is being applied in every door entering our life, it is the most absolute avenue to ensure success. Good natural light, looking only at good peaceful images when seeking healing and therapeutic responses from our bodies. Treatments in nature or in a garden become much more beneficial than the sterile typical treatment office where all-natural light is closed off.

Proper and natural foods used in conjunction with God's teachings, and in a manner that is honoring to Him thus fasting at times. Illuminating any poisons, processed foods, artificial sugars, or preservatives is a great start in the cleansing process. Goodness in the form of positive words spoken both by you and accepted as you receive the words of others, these positive creations not only fill your ears but surround your environment with goodness and Light-giving energies. Images in your eyes, good words read, beautiful images, seen, peace bathing your eyes as you fill your heart with pure Godly light.

This is the single most advantageous application therapy for treating children regardless of their afflictions. I was amazed that when these factors would be applied to children more than anyone demonstrated the most rapid and seemingly miraculous ability to overcome and heal. Children are for the most part fed this world through the parents one spoon at a time and thus have the greatest responsibility of only giving the child goodness in light, sound, words, feeding, drinking, and feeling they can so the child can in their own belief grow to experience the world in so many ways. Parent fear, any loving parent knows this, but expressing this fear to the child even out of concern is the same as reading the child's fear, and should be avoided at all costs. Warning the child of the bully only makes the child afraid and thus lures the bully to them, but empowering the child to overcome the bully that is the greatest gift a parent can give.

God Himself said; *"I would that all of you come to me as children."*

Good peaceful sounds such as calming music or soft meditation music aids in the sound department when granting a positive environment for healing, but filling the ears with nothing negative, only positive uplifting and encouraging words is key for the increase of goodness in one's life. And if success is to be guaranteed then words of forgiveness spoken and heard are instrumental for driving away spirits that may still be inflicting a person.

But remember to always forgive yourself for being a participant in the issues that have harmed you. People themselves are always their own hardest judges, forgiving others for the very things they refuse to forgive themselves for.

Good natural foods, pure natural plant products for the reduction of symptoms, natural oils for positive applications of love and care in massages, touches, and natural reflex treatments any and all of these are just a few of everything that resides around us merely to be picked up and used for the treatment of issues arising from the survival of a storm.

"A loving touch is a gift you can so freely give, and its treasure is beyond your ability to totally comprehend in this physical world."

We Are All Flowers

One of the earliest memories I had regarding a speaking word or thought from God, and writing it down, came very shortly after the first word I received, and had a marked effect on me directly and for years to come. I remember stating perhaps in my prayer and maybe even out loud to God; "So if You would that everyone would be healed, what is stopping them, why do only a few seemed to be healed?"

"What is the difference? Why do some have miracles, and some don't? Especially when they, and I, all seem to be asking?"

I asked that question, didn't get much of an answer, yet at the very moment, I asked it, in my mind an image of a beautiful Tuscan landscape came in front of my eyes, filled my vision painting a landscape with beautiful colors; reds, purples, whites, and greens, flowing winds cascading across the fields as it gently flowed in the summers breeze. A solum tree standing in the center, strong and picturesque, like a guarding sentinel protecting all under its reaching arms.

A few months later I was hiking with a nurse friend who upon hearing my story of the passing of my first wife and child in a car accident, promptly told me of her own experience of the passing of her child while still a baby.

As comforting as it was, it was rare for me to speak to someone regarding the loss of my spouse or child, or in this case both. The only people that seemed to understand, were people who went through such losses themselves, prompting me to not only talk about it with her but also to write this account very early on in my writing career.

This is from that writing;

I knew a man once, a long time ago, he was a younger man, naive yet full of faith. Faith in God but also in the world! This man always loved God, even walked and talked with Him his whole life, but often knew not how to show it.

Then one day he found himself in a far-off land, and the last thing he expected happened; God decided to bless him by allowing our young traveler to meet one of God's "Truly wonderful flowers"!

It didn't take long for this man to fall in love with the flower, because everyone who ever met her loved her. But another true miracle occurred, she actually loved him as well! Giving up school, home, family, even country, in a place that didn't speak his language, for a gift given by God didn't seem like a sacrifice at all, but more a privilege.

Days and nights filled with laughter, most of the time at nothing at all, coupled with the sweet scent of fresh dew on newly blossomed flowers, the misty morn of a cool spring day, so was her breath. A touch so soft yet graced with strength, that it lit a flame in this man's heart that encircled said heart as gently as a warm feather bed snuggles shoulders on a cold winter's night.

Every curl, every curve, every small glance, her mere touch was as perfect as the speckling of beauty marks on her legs that randomly adorned her being like the stars of the sky. Perfect, maybe not by world's standards, but to him as perfect as any glorious creation his young eyes had yet witnessed.

How sweet it was to sit across a crowded room and have her look at him, mouth a word, and he would know exactly everything she said. How sweet was it to come from a feast every day that was her, and be so full he couldn't even glance at another morsel.

She was his love, she was his heart, she was his friend, she was his life. She was his wife!

A man would risk, even sacrifice his life gladly to protect the precious pearl that God has blessed him with. She does as well; risks her own, sacrificing body, risking life to joyfully bring a child into the world.

Blessings beyond imagination!

Some would say our young traveler had it all when you have everything you need all the extras are just extra and really only amount to simple pleasures that rain down from God as simple flakes of snow in a perfect winter's scene.

But suddenly one day which should have been glorious, being only a single one before the scheduled day of birth of their second child, beauty turns to tragedy! A stranger who would rush to beat a red light would cross her path, and life for her, as well as the child, would disappear from her blue eyes.

To understand the depth of what he experienced, only those that have experienced similar losses can feel the pain, and through this common feeling, this kind of tragic experience, can one relate to what he went through after that horrific day.

When I say those of similar loss, I mean someone who has a part of themselves taken from this world. Not to diminish anyone's loss, whether it is a parent, a dear friend, or a close loved one, but nothing seems to compare to the loss of a spouse or child! This may very well be due to the fact that a child is created with a piece of ourselves. In the same way, when two people become one flesh as is the case in marriage, in some cases they become one person.

The loss of either of these kinds of individuals in our lives can leave us not only depressed at this loss but left with a sense of utter and unexplainable incompleteness. We feel like a part of us is missing, and no matter what we do, we can't seem to find a fill to that lost part!

Why he asked?!!!

Our young traveler, our angry, confused, guilt-ridden, tired young believer, would enter the wilderness! Wander with fist-in-air, kicking rocks, head down, eyes turned away from the glare of a day that has become various shades of grey.

Days turned into weeks, which turned into years. Relationships came and went, and with them came various levels of betrayal even from those who pledged thier deepest devotion.

Funny how a man can just slowly walk into a "Death Valley," slowly descending, unknowingly, most of the time, until he finds himself so far below the "Sea" level, that he can hardly imagine a way out. When all seems lost and giving up becomes something our blessed, not so young man possibly looks at for the first time in his life, finally, out of desperation, he calls out to Jesus for help, and Jesus answers! In a bathtub of all places!

The climb out is a rapid ascent when God shows us the path! Three things happen when you get to the other side, at the top of the mountain ridge that crests the edge of the valley; one, you can look back and see the whole valley, giving a clear picture of the whole and what exactly it was, and two, it doesn't look so big as it did when you were deep in, and third, a person might even thank Him for the experience of overcoming, the task won, the lesson learned!

God is so good! Not only does He rescue His child when called, but He also blesses our traveler with the answer to his "why?" question that has haunted him all the years of his wilderness walk.

One day he was asked by a female friend who had also had a tragic loss of a child. When she heard of his loss she turned, with tears in her eyes said; "If God loves as you say He does, then how do you explain the loss of an innocent person such as your wife or child, or my baby?"

At this point, our new recruit in God's army had become a "Believer" and knew Jesus lived in his heart, but the answer to that question he had never quite heard!

He closed his eyes and asked God for wisdom. God spoke in his mind. "Well, you said we could ask anything and it would be given?" "So I am asking?"

An image immediately appeared;

He softly speaks into her ear; "I just had the vision of a beautiful field of flowers, mostly reds, but also yellows, violets, and whites, appear in my mind. In the middle of a sweeping hill-lined valley meadow stood a shady tree, quite inviting and peaceful! You know the kind they show on a travel brochure to Tuscany, Italy or someplace like that?"

"Peaceful, restful, perfect in order and design, balanced majesty of symphonic grace as the breeze gently flows over blossoms, like the caressing waves of a green-tinted shore."

"Then I heard the voice of God just say in my head;"

"Consider the flowers;"

"Some lie in the middle of the field, where the Sun is strong and the soil is deep, plenty of water, safe."

"Some lie under the trees, a good safe place but not as much of the Sun, they just don't seem to grow as well."

"Some lie in the rocks, where the soil is thin and water spars, they do not grow well at all, a seemingly poor life."

"Some lie in the weeds, where life is hard and struggle seems to be a daily event, their short life choked out sometimes cruelly."

"And some lie on the road, where the wagon comes by and snuffs out their life suddenly!"

"You are all those flowers in that field! You are all flowers to me; some you are strong, some of you are weak, some of you are tall, some are small, all equal, all loved, all perfect."

"Yours is not to understand why this one lies here, or that

one there, in my most perfect field, yours is to Thank Me, for the time you got spend with my most precious flowers!"

Our young believer then understood and had an overwhelming realization that he needed to "thank God" for two things; for all the precious time he got to spend in his life with such a beautiful creation as one of God's precious flowers, his wife and even unborn child. If it was but a moment, it was infinitely better than to have never had known them at all! And two; that God loves him enough to let me see the rest of the beauty of this gift we call our life, seeing not only our place in it, but his hand in every sight, sound, taste, and breath we share. If God didn't have all of the flowers in their perfect place, and in their perfect color, we wouldn't have the even more glorious field!

The true picture of life, as He sees it, and as we experience it.

This traveler was me!

God is faithful, I have had precious time with one of His most precious flowers.

That was many years ago, praise God I have also had since been promised restoration, and God always keeps His promises.

A flower?

Could God have another for me, and allow me to be one for her!

"Yes"

About The Authors

Peter Colla, the author, is an American-born, European-trained practicing Physical Therapist, Artist, Writer, Husband, and Father. Whether it was the fact that he sustained a life-threatening infection of which he was miraculously and completely healed from, one that nearly resulted in the loss of his leg, or the fact that his father contracted MS when he just started studying medicine, he was prompted to study physical therapy, return to America, and practice for over thirty years. Recently married to Anna Colla, the Co-Author and Muse, a European born, practicing International Entertainer, Dancer, Pilates Instructor, Motivational Speaker, wife, and mother, has joined him in an east meets west examination of the spiritual elements surrounding healing. Together they form a powerful two become one team designed and empowered to demonstrate the faithful gifts all of us can enjoy when we look first to God for our healing, health, and wellness. Recently they formed GEMS of Health and Wellness to bring the many treasures, experiences, and gems of wisdom they have been so freely given to anyone who wishes to try.

Two ends of the earth, two philosophies of treatment, East meets West in this practical examination of the Body, Mind and most importantly Spirit, in the form of Belief, all seemingly missing, at least in part in today's medicine. In a conversational format with God, our authors have chronicled observations, and revelations to help individuals be free of the chains of sickness, injury, doubt, and hopelessness.

Over ten years in the making, a practicing medical physical therapist joins with a spiritually guided Pilates instructor and fine arts dancer, teaming up in the holiest union to examine the correlations between Godly healings and medical expectations of today. Both of them experiencing personal miracles of healing in their own pasts, as well as the many they have witnessed since drives them to search for the missing elements in medicine that seem to stimulate miraculous recovery in people not only in the faith environment but naturally all over the world today.

Look with us as we reexamine the factors of Body, Mind, and Spirit with simple and understandable illustrations outlining successful treatment models, and the assimilation of a workable guideline for people to use for themselves as a means for them to receive total miraculous healing, regardless of their religious or philosophical bias. This quest has put all of us on a path that allows anyone willing to open up and examine the correlation of today's medicine, with the more physical therapy like, as well as natural holistic healing arts demonstrated and documented nearly two thousand years ago by the man who no one doubts to be the most successful healer in the history of the world; Jesus.

Disclaimer

The disclaimer provides that such medical information is merely information and not advice. If users need medical advice, they should consult a doctor or other appropriate medical professional. The disclaimer also provides that no warranties are given in relation to the medical information supplied on the website and that no liability will occur to the website owner in the event that a user suffers loss as a result of reliance upon the information. All content found in this book, Gems of Health and Wellness, GEM Village websites, paulorpeter.com, affiliates, or published materials, including text, images, audio, or other formats were created for informational purposes only. Offerings for education, public speaking, and seminars are clearly identified and the appropriate target audience is identified. The Content is not intended to be a substitute for professional medical advice, diagnosis, or treatment. Always seek the advice of your physician or other qualified health providers with any questions you may have regarding a medical condition. Never disregard professional medical advice or delay in seeking it because of something you have read or heard in this material.

If you think you may have a medical emergency, call your doctor, go to the emergency department, or call 911 immediately. Peter and Anna Colla do not recommend or endorse any specific tests, physicians, products, procedures, opinions, or other information that may be mentioned in the Gems of Health and Wellness material. Reliance on any information provided by gems-of-health-and-wellness.com, Gem Village employees, contracted writers, or medical professionals presenting content for publication to this book or any other material associated with Peter and Anna Colla is solely at your own risk. The writings, materials, or websites may contain health or medical-related materials or discussions regarding sexually explicit disease states. If you find these materials offensive, you may not want to use our material. The Book, Web Site, published material, and or it's Content are provided on an "as is" basis. Links to educational and reference content not created by Peter and Anna Colla are taken at your own risk. Peter and Anna Colla and Gems of Health and Wellness are not responsible for the claims of external websites and education companies.

Peter Colla

Made in the USA
Columbia, SC
17 September 2021